Dermatologic
Surgery Tips and
Techniques

Commissioning Editor: **Karen Bowler**
Development Editor: **Cecilia Murphy**
Editorial Assistant: **Nani Clansey**
Project Manager: **Alan Nicholson**
Design: **Andy Chapman**
Illustration Manager: **Bruce Hogarth**
Marketing Managers: **Clara Toombs (UK) and Lisa Damico (USA)**

Dermatologic Surgery Tips and Techniques

Stuart J. Salasche MD
Clinical Professor
University of Arizona Health Sciences Center
Tucson AZ
USA

Ida F. Orengo MD
Director of Dermatologic Surgery
Professor of Dermatology
Department of Dermatology
Baylor College of Medicine
Houston TX
USA

Ronald J. Siegle MD
Clinical Professor of Dermatology
and Clinical Professor of Otolaryngology, Head and Neck Surgery
Ohio State University College of Medicine
Columbus OH
USA

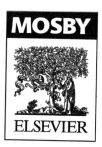

MOSBY

ELSEVIER

MOSBY
ELSEVIER

Mosby is an affiliate of Elsevier Inc.

© 2007, Elsevier Inc. All rights reserved.

First published 2007

ISBN-13: 978-0-323-03462-3
ISBN-10: 0-323-03462-4

British Library Cataloguing in Publication Data
A catalogue record for this book is available from the British Library

Library of Congress Cataloging in Publication Data
A catalog record for this book is available from the Library of Congress

---

Notice
Medical knowledge is constantly changing. Standard safety precautions must be followed, but as new research and clinical experience broaden our knowledge, changes in treatment and drug therapy may become necessary or appropriate. Readers are advised to check the most current product information provided by the manufacturer of each drug to be administered to verify the recommended dose, the method and duration of administration, and contraindications. It is the responsibility of the practitioner, relying on experience and knowledge of the patient, to determine dosages and the best treatment for each individual patient. Neither the Publisher nor the author assume any liability for any injury and/or damage to persons or property arising from this publication.
The Publisher

Printed and bound by CPI Group (UK) Ltd, Croydon, CR0 4YY

Transferred to digital print 2012

Contents

Contents

Acknowledgments

The authors would like to acknowledge the following contributors:

Daniel Zivony, MD, co-author of the chapters on Flaps and Grafts in Sections 4 and 5.

Suneel Chilukuri, who contributed several Tips in Section 7 on Instruments.

Dedication

I dedicate this book to my wife, Jan.

Stuart J. Salasche

I dedicate this book with love to my husband Ed, a great soccer dad and take-out chef; to my wonderful children, Sarah, Matthew, Anna, and Jacob, who charm and motivate my days and gave me permission to type at night; and to my parents, Antonio and Cristina, who made it all possible by teaching me to learn, to think and to write.

Ida F. Orengo

As an academic dermatologic surgeon, I wrote multiple articles and chapters, just as my good friends and colleagues did (Neil, Shelly, Stu, and so many more). As the years went by, the one missing piece, from a publishing point of view, was a textbook. There were two driving forces for me to write a book. The first was academic fulfilment. The second was so that I could proclaim publicly and in print on a dedication page my enormous (profound, unending, indescribable) thanks to several very special people.

To Marian and Mannie, I could not have had better parents. Your love, support and guidance was and still is always there. I could ask for nothing more. I owe you everything.

To my wife Ruthie, my best friend, thank you for your endless support, understanding and guidance over all of these years. It has been a wonderful journey that would not have occurred without you.

To my children Gabe and Hannah, who make me so proud, thank you for your patience and understanding as I followed my passion. I wish the same for you.

To you all, I dedicate this book.

With all my love,

Ron (Dad)

Ronald J. Siegle

Section 1
Assisting at surgery

TIP 1
Surgical Assistant
Counter-Traction and a Clear Visual Field

 Rationale:

- A properly trained surgical assistant (SA) makes surgery more efficient and safer.
- The surgeon is responsible for the education and training of the surgical assistant so that duties, responsibilities, the surgical plan and the surgeon's routine are clear.
- This includes professional deportment in the outpatient operating room where patients are awake, alert and apprehensive.
- Among the various duties of the surgical assistant are maintaining a clear visual surgical field and providing counter-traction.

 Technique:

- The SA should always be 'doing something,' even if it is just anticipating what needs to be done next.
- The SA should have at least '4 hands' and have all the 'next' instruments ready to go (*Fig. 1.1*).
- There should always be a 4 × 4 gauze sponge in each hand for blotting blood and providing firm, non-distorting counter-traction creating a clear visual field (*Fig. 1.2*).
- The gauze works better than gloved fingers, which become slippery with blood.
- The SA is instructed not to make sudden changes in traction; if blood is welling up in the field, the SA should ask for cutting to stop before blotting the wound (*Fig. 1.3*).
- Counter-traction for the second limb of an elliptical incision or circular excision can be achieved by the SA grasping and retracting the already cut edge of the tissue laterally with a toothed forceps or cotton-tipped applicator (*Figs 1.4 and 1.5*).

 Advantage:

- An SA who understands the surgical plan and anticipates the needs of the surgeon makes surgery much more efficient.

 Reference:

Salasche SJ, Winton GB, Adnot J. Surgical pearls. Dermatol Clin 1989; 7:75–110.

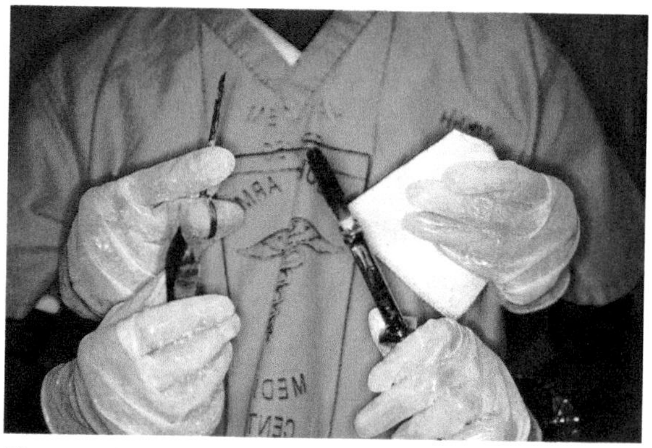

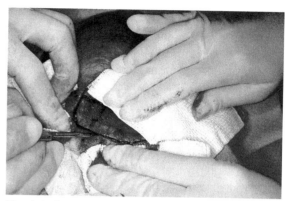

Fig. 1.1 The surgical assistant can perform many tasks.

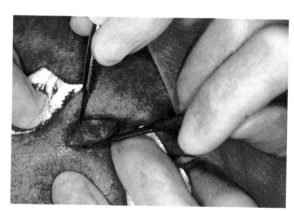

Fig. 1.2 Counter-traction and a clear visual field.

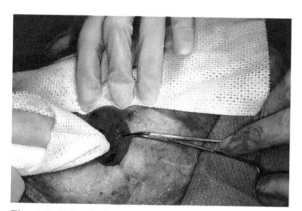

Fig. 1.3 Aiding in hemostasis.

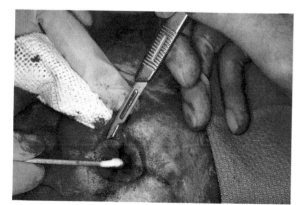

Fig. 1.4 Counter-traction with a forceps.

Fig. 1.5 Counter-traction and stabilization with a cotton-tipped applicator.

Rationale:

- The simple interrupted stitch is the entry-level technique for closing wounds of the skin.
- It is also used to initiate most surface running sutures.
- Conquering the principles of this stitch gives the budding surgeon a solid base for learning more complicated suturing techniques.
- It is best learned as a repetitive exercise with each component having a fixed method of performance.
- The key is to create a flask-shaped design with the deeper portion being slightly wider than the surface bites.
- When this is done correctly, the skin edges are gently coapted and everted.
- It reinforces and refines the work done by the buried vertical subcuticular stitches that classically precede placement of the surface stitches.

Technique:

- Begin on the side of the wound furthest away (far side) from the surgeon.
- Insure the initial insertion of the needle is about 2–3 mm from the wound edge and is either perpendicular (90 degrees) to the skin surface (Fig. 2.1) or slightly directed away from the wound for even greater eversion.
- Continuation of this arc naturally creates a wider bite at the lower portion of the wound (Fig. 2.2).
- This exit point is not in the wound edge, but rather below the entry point where the skin was undermined (Fig. 2.2).
- It is best to 'show the point' in the center of the wound before attempting to re-enter the deep portion of the skin.
- Enter the near side equidistant from the exit point, again entering at a 90-degree angle (Fig. 2.3).
- Continuing the natural curve of the arc of the needle will cause the needle to exit the skin at the same distance from the wound edge as the original entry point (Fig. 2.4).
- When tied off, the edges will be everted (Fig. 2.5).

Advantage:

- The advantageous eversion will settle down during the ensuing weeks and a scar flush with the surface will be cosmetically pleasing.

Caveat:

- The usual error is to enter the skin at a 'skimming' angle that will produce a shallow bite and inability to yield the desired eversion (Fig. 2.6).

Reference:

Fewkes JL, Cheney ML, Pollack SV, eds. Illustrated atlas of cutaneous surgery. Philadelphia: JB Lippincott; 1992:11.2–11.4.

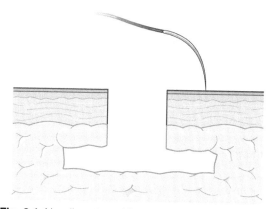

Fig. 2.1 Needle enters skin at 90 degrees.

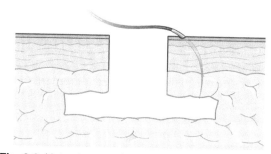

Fig. 2.2 Natural curve of needle creates wider defect at bottom.

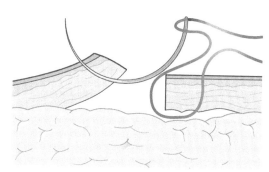

Fig. 2.3 Re-entry equidistant will create symmetric curved pass.

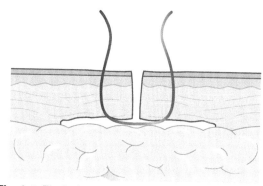

Fig. 2.4 Flask-shaped suture track.

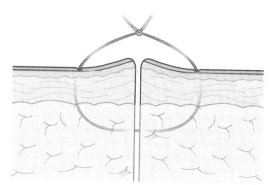

Fig. 2.5 Eversion created when tied off.

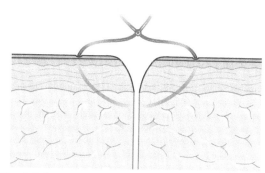

Fig. 2.6 Incorrect placement at shallow angle causes inversion.

TIP 3
Surgical Assistant
Help with Surface Sutures

 Rationale:

- Simple interrupted, vertical mattress and the various running stitches constitute the mainstay 'finishing' suturing techniques used to complete a surgical closure, be it a side-to-side closure, flap or graft.
- The surgeon may either bring the needle out within the suture line or pass it all the way through both sides of the wound edge in a single pass.
- Depending on the needle size, the extent of the bite and the thickness of the skin, this may prove difficult and is facilitated by a surgical assistant (SA).

 Technique:

- Whether the needle is brought out in the suture line or passed through both wound edges, the SA can help secure the needle tip below the point with a toothless forceps (*Fig. 3.1*).
- The SA then guides the needle out of the skin where it is held in position for the surgeon to re-grasp it with the needle holder (*Fig. 3.2*).
- If the needle tip encounters resistance in passing up through to the surface of the skin, the SA presses down around the needle-induced protuberance with an open toothed forceps until the point pops up (*Figs 3.3, 3.4 and 3.5*).
- It is then grasped below the point and rotated out (*Fig. 3.6*).

 Advantage:

- Needle point is handled with instruments, not fingers.
- Less likely to bend the needle.

 Caveat:

- Don't grasp needle point, it will dull it.
- Keeps fingers out of the field.

 Variant:

- Surgeon may push down with non-dominant hand to provide counter-traction and allow needle to pop through skin.

 Reference:

Salasche SJ, Winton GB, Adnot J. Surgical pearls. Dermatol Clin 1989; 7:75–110.

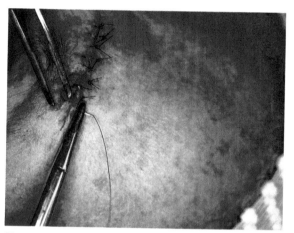

Fig. 3.1 SA grasps needle as it protrudes through skin. (From Salasche SJ, Winton GB, Adnot J. Surgical Pearls. Dermatol Clin 1989; 7:75–110.)

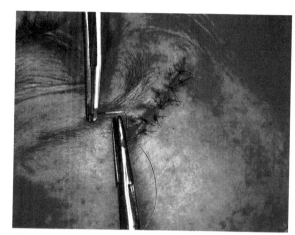

Fig. 3.2 SA rotates out needle and holds for re-grasping. (From Salasche SJ, Winton GB, Adnot J. Surgical Pearls. Dermatol Clin 1989; 7:75–110.)

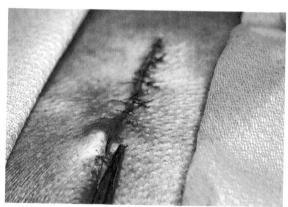

Fig. 3.3 Needle can't penetrate skin. (From Salasche SJ, Winton GB, Adnot J. Surgical Pearls. Dermatol Clin 1989; 7:75–110.)

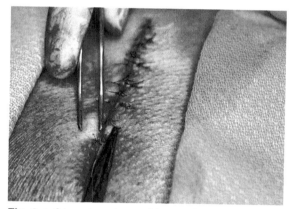

Fig. 3.4 SA pushes down with open forceps. (From Salasche SJ, Winton GB, Adnot J. Surgical Pearls. Dermatol Clin 1989; 7:75–110.)

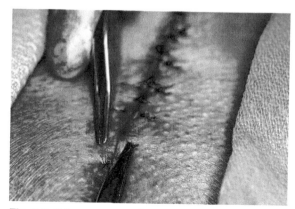

Fig. 3.5 SA secures needle as it pops through.

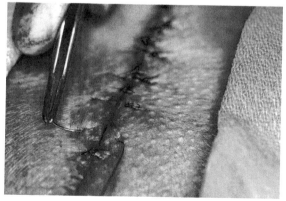

Fig. 3.6 Needle rotated out of skin. (From Salasche SJ, Winton GB, Adnot J. Surgical Pearls. Dermatol Clin 1989; 7:75–110.)

Surgical Assistant
Twisted Knot and Cutting Suture at Correct Length

 Rationale:
- The vertical mattress stitch requires passing the suture material back and forth and the thread may become kinked when attempting to tie the knot.
- Another problem is cutting the suture at the proper length after a knot is secured. A well-known lament from the surgical assistant (SA) cliché goes: 'Doctor, do you want me to cut them long or short today?'

 Technique:
- When placing the vertical mattress stitch, it may become twisted, tangled or kinked when securing the initial double throw (*Fig. 4.1*).
- A twisted knot will not tie properly.
- The SA can insert the closed prongs of the toothless forceps (or other instrument) and straighten out the kink by opening the blades (*Fig. 4.2*).
- The surgeon can close the loop around the forceps which are slipped out as the knot is tightened across the suture line.
- A simple way to always have sutures cut at the appropriate length is to crisscross them where you wish them snipped (*Fig. 4.3*).
- The suture is snipped where the strands intersect (*Fig. 4.4*).
- The suture is cut at the correct length (*Fig. 4.5*).

 Advantage:
- Foolproof method for cutting suture; eliminates guilt and anger.

 Caveat:
- Hold crossing point of strings steady until snipping is accomplished.

 Reference:
Salasche SJ, Winton GB, Adnot J. Surgical pearls. Dermatol Clin 1989; 7:75–110.

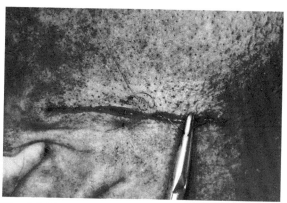

Fig. 4.1 Mattress suture: twisted initial double throw won't lie down properly. (From Salasche SJ, Winton GB, Adnot J. Surgical Pearls. Dermatol Clin 1989; 7:75–110.)

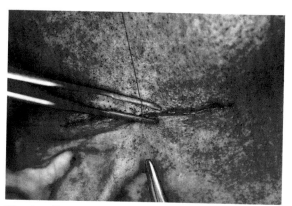

Fig. 4.2 Forceps corrects the kink in knot. (From Salasche SJ, Winton GB, Adnot J. Surgical Pearls. Dermatol Clin 1989; 7:75–110.)

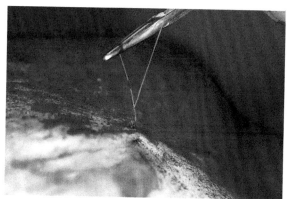

Fig. 4.3 Cross strands where sutures are to be cut. (From Salasche SJ, Winton GB, Adnot J. Surgical Pearls. Dermatol Clin 1989; 7:75–110.)

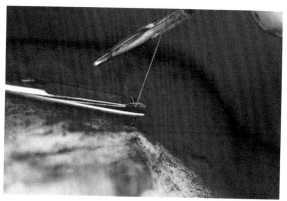

Fig. 4.4 Sutures cut. (From Salasche SJ, Winton GB, Adnot J. Surgical Pearls. Dermatol Clin 1989; 7:75–110.)

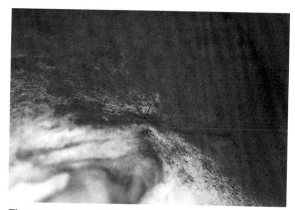

Fig. 4.5 Appropriate length.

TIP 5
Surgical Assistant
Help with the Buried Subcuticular Stitch

Rationale:

- During surgery there are simple, repetitive events related to closure and suturing where the surgical assistant (SA) can be of great help.
- It is much more efficient to place subcuticular stitches with the aid of an experienced SA, who can help in several points throughout the procedure.

Technique:

- The SA can help with needle transfer similar to when assisting on surface sutures described in Tip 3.
- This entails maintaining good field exposure and finger-free placement and transfer of the needle.
- An important function is keeping a vigil to make sure the strands are on the same side and not on opposite sides of the central horizontal thread (*Fig. 5.1*).
- After the first pass, the SA should grasp the long non-needle end of the suture and hold it visibly to one side or the other so the surgeon can easily see it and then remove the needle from the wound on the same side.
- If they are on opposite sides, the knot will lock before all the slack is gone and a gap in the wound will result (*Fig. 5.2*).
- The SA can assist in adjusting the suture strands so that they remain on the same side by reaching under the cross-strand and pulling one errant side to the same side (*Figs 5.3 and 5.4*).
- Assistance can also be rendered in placing the knot.
- As the surgeon snugs down the initial double surgeon's throw, the SA compresses the wound edges together until the knot is secured at the base of the wound (*Fig. 5.5*).
- After all the knots are thrown, the surgeon holds the suture strands up to expose the knot.
- The SA slides the cutting scissors down to the knot, rotates the scissors about 15–30 degrees, and snips (*Fig. 5.6*).
- If the subcuticular stitch has been properly placed, the knot will then retract down to the lowest portion of the wound.

Advantages:

- Ensures strands are on same side; if opposite sides, knot won't tie properly.
- Without an SA to take tension off the wound edges, there may be some slack in the subcuticular stitch.
- If there is slack, after the knots are tied there may be a gap in the wound suture line.

Reference:
Salasche SJ, Winton GB, Adnot J. Surgical pearls. Dermatol Clin 1989; 7:75–110.

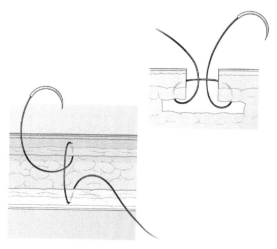

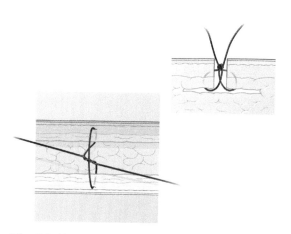

Fig. 5.1 Proper subcuticular stitch design, but strands on opposite sides of central horizontal thread.

Fig. 5.2 Knot locks before all slack is taken up.

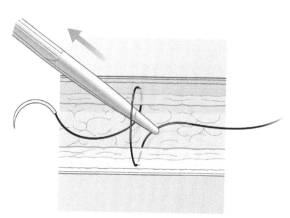

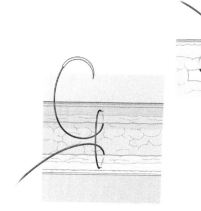

Fig. 5.3 Errant strand pulled into place on same side.

Fig. 5.4 Suture on same side.

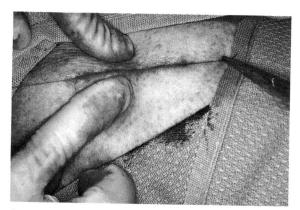

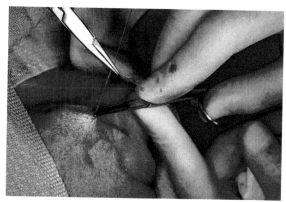

Fig. 5.5 SA compresses wound edges.

Fig. 5.6 Cutting buried suture just above knot.

Section **2**
Suture techniques

How to Break the Memory of Suture Material without Breaking the Suture

Rationale:

- Some suture materials, such as the popular Prolene (polypropylene), possess a considerable amount of memory.
- Memory is the tendency of the suture material to return to its original shape after being deformed.
- This is manifested by the strand retaining its many loops after being removed from the package (*Fig. 6.1*).
- These loops get in the way and hinder placement of both deep and surface sutures.
- This is particularly bothersome when performing one of the continuous or running sutures.
- Memory can also adversely affect knot security if the suture is not properly tied with alternating reverse square knots.

Technique:

- A simple technique to break the memory is to grasp the thread with the thumb and index finger of one hand just beyond the swaged-on insertion of the suture material into the hollowed-out and then crimped needle shank.
- As the thread is held firmly, it is drawn through the compressing index finger and thumb of the other hand (*Fig. 6.2*).
- If the swaged-on connection to the needle shank is not protected, the suture can be pulled out, wasting the whole packet (*Figs 6.3, 6.4 and 6.5*).
- Another related tip, which one would think is obvious, is to open the suture packet where indicated.
- Many beginners just rip anywhere along the packet when opening, and have trouble locating the needle.
- If opened as directed, the needle comes immediately into view and in position to be grasped easily and safely by the needle driver (*Fig. 6.6*).
- Yet another tip is to actually read the packet; it contains much valuable information on size/type of needle and color/length/thickness of the thread and may prevent opening an incorrect suture (*Fig. 6.2*).

Advantage:

- Makes difficult-to-use suture material more pliable.

Caveat:

- Avoid pulling the swaged-on strand out of the needle: expensive.

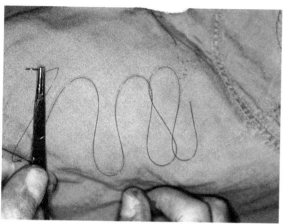

Fig. 6.1 Strand of Prolene coils indicating high memory.

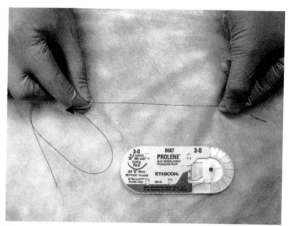

Fig. 6.2 Correct method of breaking memory.

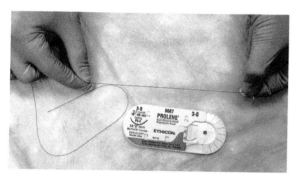

Fig. 6.3 Incorrect technique: holding needle with fingers.

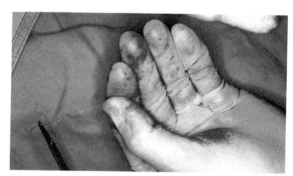

Fig. 6.4 Incorrect technique: holding needle with needle holder.

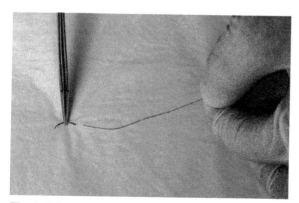

Fig. 6.5 Strand pulled out of needle.

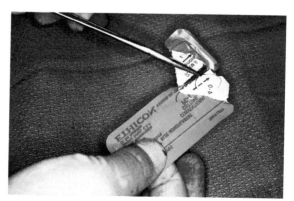

Fig. 6.6 Needle exposed and safely removed with needle holder.

TIP 7
Hemostasis
Suture Ligature

Rationale:

- Hemostasis is usually achieved with combinations of pressure, electrosurgery of various types, or topical chemical agents.
- Periodically, there is brisk bleeding from visible vessels >1 mm in diameter.
- Sometimes an exposed vessel is visible, but not bleeding.
- In this case, the vessel may have been nicked but, because of epinephrine in the anesthetic fluid or natural vasoconstriction, bleeding is not evident, but may occur later.
- Both of these instances are indications for suture ligature.

Technique:

- There are two common techniques, the stick-tie and the figure-of-eight tie.
- The stick-tie is appropriate when the exposed vessel is visible and pointing upward and vertical.
- Initially, the exposed end of the vessel is grasped with a fine, angulated hemostat (*Fig.7.1*).
- A small bite of tissue is taken behind the hemostat (*Fig. 7.2*).
- The suture is then tied off in front of the hemostat to include the vessel (*Fig. 7.3*).
- The hemostat is removed as the first knot is snugged down.
- This effectively closes off the vessel.
- Appropriately sized absorbable suture such as 5:0 Vicryl (polyglactin) should be used.
- The suture is cut short just above the knot so as to not leave excessive string in the wound (*Fig. 7.4*).

- The figure-of-eight tie is appropriate when the bleeding vessel does not extend above the wound bed surface.
- The bleeder is again grasped with a fine, angulated hemostat.
- Care is taken not to gather up much surrounding tissue.
- An angled bite is taken on one side of the bleeder (*Figs 7.5 and 7.6*).
- It is then brought out and a second angled bite is taken on the other side, as indicated in *Figure 7.7*.
- When tying off, the hemostat is again removed as the first knot is snugged down.
- The vessel is effectively surrounded and it collapses as the suture is tied (*Fig. 7.8*).

Advantage:

- Successful suture ligature of appropriate vessels mitigates late bleeding and hematoma formation.

Caveats:

- Make sure vessel is secured within the tie.
- Avoid gathering up too much normal tissue; only a secure anchoring bite is required.

Reference:

Billingsley EM, Maloney ME. Considerations in achieving hemostasis. In: Robinson JK, Arndt KA, et al., eds. Atlas of cutaneous surgery. Philadelphia: WB Saunders; 1996:69–71.

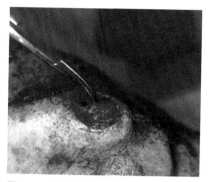

Fig. 7.1 Exposed vessel grasped with a fine, angulated hemostat.

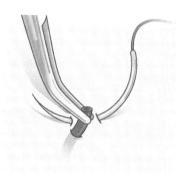

Fig. 7.2 A bite is taken behind the hemostat.

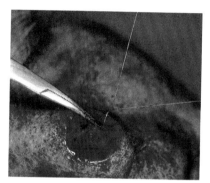

Fig. 7.3 The stick-tie is secure and ready to be tied off.

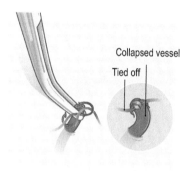

Fig. 7.4 Vessel collapses as suture tied.

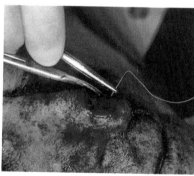

Fig. 7.5 Initial bite of a figure-of-eight ligature.

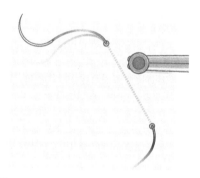

Fig. 7.6 Diagram of initial bite.

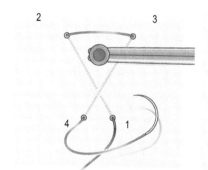

Fig. 7.7 Diagram of sequence of bites for figure-of-eight ligature.

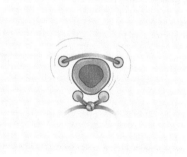

Fig. 7.8 Vessel collapses as suture is tied off.

Proper Placement of the Three-Cornered Stitch

Rationale:

- The three-cornered stitch is often used to secure the apex of an M-plasty or a V-Y closure.
- Improper placement is common, resulting in inadequate 'seating' or inset of the apex fully into the 'V.'
- Improper placement of the tip stitch may also result in necrosis of the tip.
- The usual error is to place the three-cornered stitch too close to the 'V' inset (*Figs 8.1 and 8.2*).

Technique:

- Start the first entry point several millimeters down the suture line beyond the apex of the 'V' (*Fig. 8.3*).
- At this point, enter the skin at 90 degrees to the surface and exit mid- to lower dermis.
- Stabilize and expose the tip by holding it loosely between the jaws of the forceps.
- Then place an arced completely buried horizontal suture at the same dermal depth as the suture exited the dermis on the initial bite (*Fig. 8.4*).
- Run the suture out of the skin opposite the initial entry point, again inserting it at the same depth in the dermis (*Figs 8.4 and 8.5*).
- Now all three points should be at the same depth within the dermis.
- Equally important is that when the stitch is tied, the tip will be pulled into place (*Fig. 8.6*).
- Snug the stitch into place using only enough tension to properly seat the apex.

Advantage:

- Gives the operator the flexibility to be able to 'pull' the apex into place without compromising the blood flow to it.

Caveats:

- Be sure there is a sufficient bite to the half-buried tip stitch.
- It shouldn't tear when pulled into place.

Variants:

- A vertical mattress tip stitch has been described with two important elements.

- The far–far initial bites should be beyond the tip inset point as described above.
- The near–near portion should include the tip via a buried bite.

References:

Starr J. Surgical tip: the vertical mattress tip stitch. J Am Acad Dermatol 2001; 44:523–524.

Bennett RG, ed. Fundamentals of cutaneous surgery. Chapter 11: Alternative suturing techniques. St. Louis: CV Mosby; 1988:458–459.

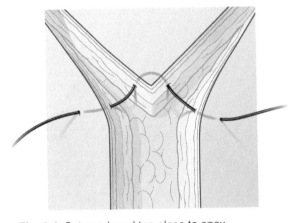

Fig. 8.1 Suture placed too close to apex.

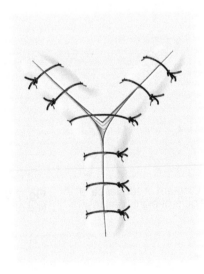

Fig. 8.2 Apex stitch when pulled into place, leaves gap and may strangle tip because it was not placed distal to the apex.

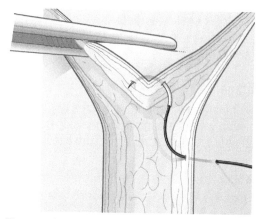

Fig. 8.3 Correct placement: transverse buried tip stitch.

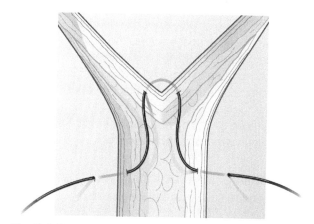

Fig. 8.4 Correct placement of all the bites.

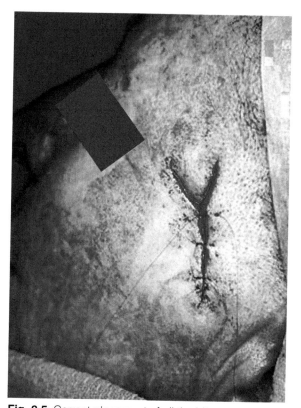

Fig. 8.5 Correct placement of all the bites.

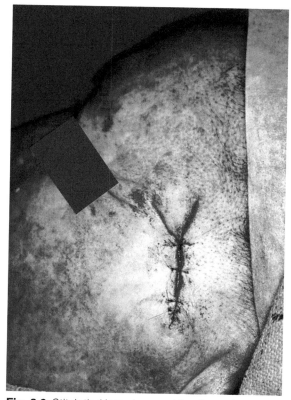

Fig. 8.6 Stitch tied into place and tip aligns nicely.

Delayed Closure of Buried Sutures When Closing Small Excisions

 Rationale:

- When closing small, especially deep excisions, limited working space makes the proper placement of buried sutures difficult.
- The tying of each buried suture further limits the space available for the placement of subsequent buried sutures.
- A variation on buried suture placement knot tying can overcome this difficulty.

 Technique:

- The buried sutures are placed in the appropriate manner throughout the wound, but left untied (*Fig. 9.1*).
- The ends of each suture are left long enough so that an instrument tie can be performed later.
- The free ends of each suture are clamped with a hemostat or taped to the surgical draping sequentially to keep them in order and out of the way from further buried suture placement (*Fig. 9.1*).
- After the desired number of sutures is placed, the individual knots are tied using standard instrument-tie technique (*Fig. 9.2*).
- It is usually best to tie the sutures closest to the apices first and work sequentially toward the center to minimize tension.

- This technique is particularly advantageous on the scalp where large needles are often required for small deep defects (*Figs 9.3, 9.4, 9.5 and 9.6*).

 Advantage:

- Proper placement of buried sutures is achieved without traumatizing the skin edges in an attempt to gain access to the site.

 Caveats:

- If adequate attention is not given to keeping each suture's two free ends together, the sutures can become tangled, making this a cumbersome technique.
- Leave sufficient string length on each suture to ensure it can be tied easily with an instrument tie.
- Will usually add an additional expense for extra suture material.

 References:

Ramsey ML, Marks VJ, Neltner SA. Surgical tip: delayed knot placement facilitates small wound closure. J Am Acad Dermatol 1996; 34:137–138.

Salasche SJ, Winton GB, Adnot J. Surgical pearls. Dermatol Clin 1989; 7:75–110.

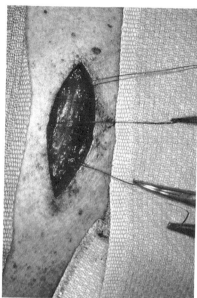

Fig. 9.1 Multiple deep sutures individually separated and secured by hemostats. (From Salasche SJ, Winton GB, Adnot J. Surgical pearls. Dermatol Clin 1989; 7:75–110.)

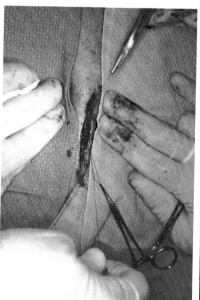

Fig. 9.2 Sequential instrument tie toward the center with help from assistant. (From Salasche SJ, Winton GB, Adnot J. Surgical pearls. Dermatol Clin 1989; 7:75–110.)

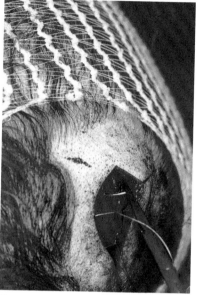

Fig. 9.3 Small, deep scalp defect; placement of deep sutures with large needle. (From Salasche SJ, Winton GB, Adnot J. Surgical pearls. Dermatol Clin 1989; 7:75–110.)

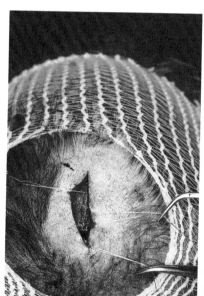

Fig. 9.4 Suture ends secured by hemostats.

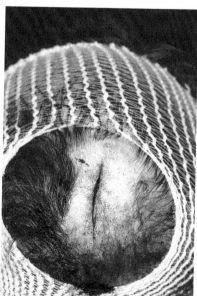

Fig. 9.5 All deep sutures tied off.

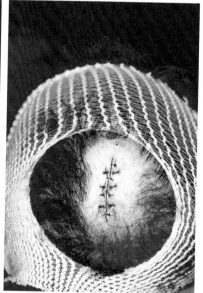

Fig. 9.6 Placement of surface sutures to complete the repair.

Percutaneous Buried Vertical Mattress Suture

Rationale:

- Placement of buried sutures is difficult in certain wounds that are deep, but short in length or where the dermis is thin.
- Sometimes the situation arises where the wound is initially closed off with deep buried vertical mattress sutures but a small, deep gap remains that would benefit from an additional suture.
- A modified buried vertical mattress suture is helpful in these situations and also offers some increased wound closure strength.

Technique:

- Upon completion of adequate undermining, the needle is inserted into the wound beginning in the deep reticular dermis or subcutis as per standard buried vertical mattress suture placement (*Fig. 10.1*).
- The needle, instead of just reaching to the high dermis and then turning back toward the wound, is actually exited through the skin surface several millimeters (3–6 mm) from the wound margin (*Fig. 10.1*).
- The needle is then reinserted into the same exit site of the skin and then quickly angled to pass through the superficial dermis and out the wound edge into the defect at the level of the reticular dermis (*Fig. 10.2*).
- These steps are repeated on the opposite side of the defect with care taken to make the height of needle entry, the bite size and the depth of needle exit the same as on the initial side (*Fig. 10.3*).
- The knot is tied in normal fashion (*Fig. 10.4*).

Advantages:

- For small wounds with limited access to the deep space, this suture is easy to place and still offers excellent eversion.
- For wounds with thin dermis and therefore a limited area to pass the needle with a traditional buried vertical mattress suture, this variation allows utilization of the full thickness of dermis and therefore increased wound strength at time of closure.

Caveats:

- The high dermal placement leaves potential for the sutures to spit at a later date.
- The suture may be torn by the needle when it is reinserted.

Reference:

Collins SC, Whalen JD. Surgical tip: percutaneous buried vertical mattress suture for the closure of narrow wounds. J Am Acad Dermatol 1999; 41:1025–1026.

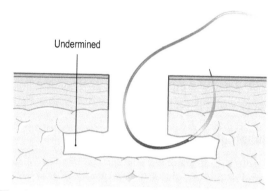

Fig. 10.1 Deep entry into subcutaneous fat or deep reticular dermis and vertical exit through skin surface.

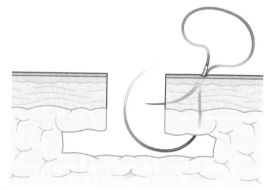

Fig. 10.2 Reinsertion of needle into same orifice and exit in mid-reticular dermis.

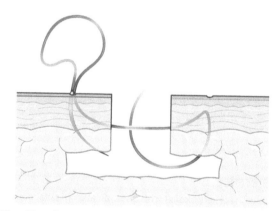

Fig. 10.3 Reverse steps on opposite side.

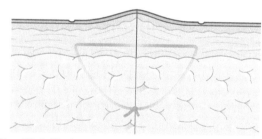

Fig. 10.4 Final tie closes dead space and everts wound edges.

Rationale:

- Because of the risk of various clotting complications when patients are taken off their anticoagulants, surgeries are being performed more frequently while patients are still taking these blood-thinning agents.
- Because of the increased risk for intraoperative and postoperative hemorrhage, certain suturing techniques have advantages over others to help minimize this risk.
- In addition, in certain locations such as the scalp, postoperative pressure dressings might be difficult to apply, resulting in problematic postoperative oozing.
- The running locked suture (also known as the baseball stitch) is a variation on the running epidermal suture, but offers greater hemostasis.

Technique:

- The initial suture is placed in a manner similar to that for a standard running suture (*Fig. 11.1*).
- Prior to beginning the second pass, the needle is passed under the loop of the suture, locking it into place (*Fig. 11.2*).
- Each successive stitch is 'locked' in a similar manner by passing the stitch under the loop before snugging it up (*Fig. 11.3*).
- Assistants are particularly helpful by holding sufficient tension on the line to keep the suture

'locked' without slack while the surgeon places the next bite (*Figs 11.4 and 11.5*).
- This is continued to the end of the incision line with the last suture tied in a standard fashion, not passing under the loop (*Fig. 11.6*).
- Coordination between the surgeon and a trained assistant helps facilitate the speed and safety of this technique.

Advantage:

- This is a strong suture which, because of the rectangular configuration of each locked unit, provides even compression and increased hemostasis along the dermal closure.

Caveats:

- The more deeply the needle is placed with each pass into the dermis, the greater the hemostasis benefit.
- Because of the compressing effect of this locking stitch, care should be taken to avoid securing it too tightly, possibly causing tissue strangulation.
- This stitch should not be used in areas of poor vascularity.

Reference:

Swanson NA, ed. Basic techniques: an atlas of cutaneous surgery. Toronto: Little Brown; 1987:44–45.

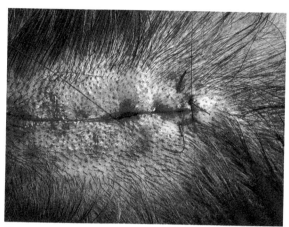

Fig. 11.1 After a simple interrupted suture the needle is brought up through the loop of the next bite.

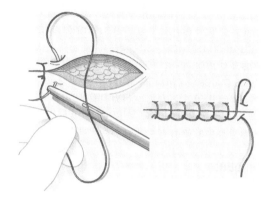

Fig. 11.2 Needle passed up through lax loop.

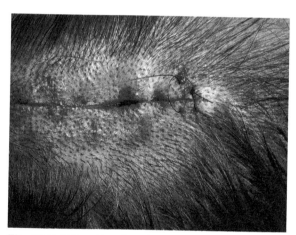

Fig. 11.3 Without tension, the loop remains loose.

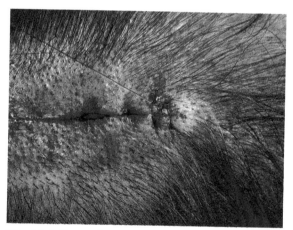

Fig. 11.4 The assistant pulls on the long end of the suture to 'lock' the suture in place.

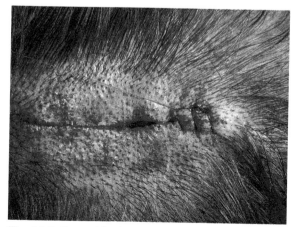

Fig. 11.5 Several 'locked loops' in place.

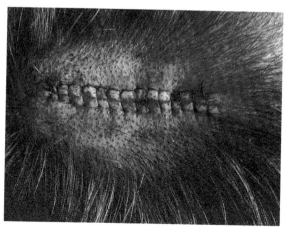

Fig. 11.6 Completed running vertical mattress stitch.

Maximal Skin Edge Eversion with the Running Hybrid Mattress Suture

Rationale:

- Tension-free skin edge eversion should be the goal for most closures as it allows the best ultimate appearance as scar maturation occurs.
- Proper dermal placement of buried sutures initiates the process and is critical to wound edge eversion.
- Where esthetic closure is paramount, simple modifications in epidermal suturing can supplement buried sutures and achieve even greater wound edge eversion.

Technique:

- Non-absorbable or fast absorbing epidermal sutures may be used.
- A simple interrupted suture is placed to start the closure (*Fig. 12.1*).
- Next, several millimeters away, a far–far bite is placed as if one were placing a traditional vertical mattress suture (*Fig. 12.1*).
- Unlike in the traditional vertical mattress where the near–near bite is taken in the same vertical axis as the far–far bite, with this technique, the needle is advanced several millimeters further along the closure line before the near–near bite is taken (*Fig. 12.2*).
- As this is a running suture, the next bite is placed several additional millimeters along the closure line and is a second far–far bite (*Fig. 12.3*).
- Alternating near–near and far–far bites are repeated until the closure is complete (*Figs 12.4 and 12.5*).

Advantages:

- This is a very easily placed suture.
- Excellent skin edge eversion is achieved.

Caveats:

- The suture should be snug, but not tight, as postoperative edema may make suture removal difficult the following week.
- The sutures should be removed by someone who is familiar with this particular suture so that small suture fragments are not left within the wound.

Reference:

Hoffman MD, Bielinski KB. Surgical tip: the hybrid mattress suture. J Am Acad Dermatol 1997; 37:773–774.

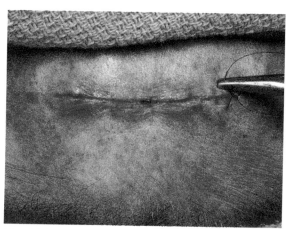

Fig. 12.1 A simple interrupted suture is placed and then several millimeters along the closure line, a slightly wider pass of the needle is made through the wound: the 'far–far' bite.

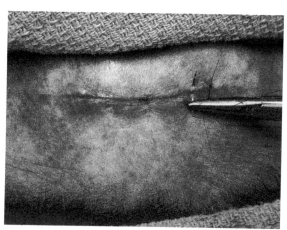

Fig. 12.2 After advancing several more millimeters, the 'near–near' pass is made entering from the same side as the far–far bite exited from.

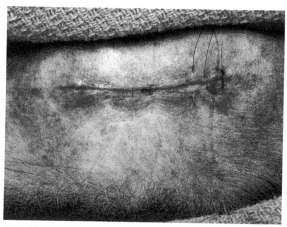

Fig. 12.3 The second 'far–far' bite.

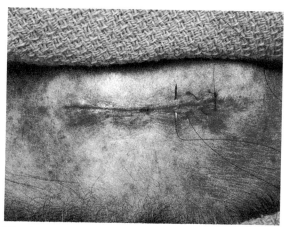

Fig. 12.4 The second 'near–near' bite.

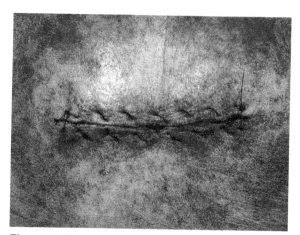

Fig. 12.5 Closure completed with alternating bites.

The Short-String Tie Off

Rationale:

- The situation often arises in which the suture string becomes short.
- The question is whether or not there is enough string for the next, and possibly the last, required stitch.
- It is expensive to open a new suture pack for one stitch.
- There is also a safety risk if the needle is manipulated by fingers under such circumstances.

Technique:

- Place the suture in the usual manner, leaving the free end as short as possible.
- Grasp the needle with an non-toothed forceps (*Fig. 13.1*).
- With the needle thus secured, loop the remaining string around the tip of the needle holder (*Fig. 13.2*).
- An initial double surgeon's throw is best, but a single loop will suffice if a square knot is formed.
- Then slightly open the needle holder and grasp the free end of the suture (*Figs 13.2 and 13.3*).
- Finally, guide it over to form the knot (*Fig. 13.4*).
- This is repeated until sufficient throws are made to secure the knot (*Fig. 13.5*).

Advantage:

- The benefits are saving the cost of opening a new suture pack and the safety of the surgeon.

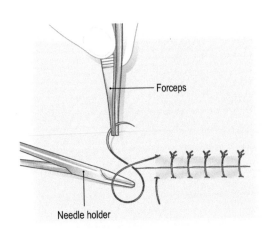

Fig. 13.1 Short-string suture with needle secured by non-toothed forceps.

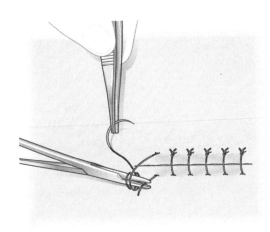

Fig. 13.2 Forming the loops around the needle holder.

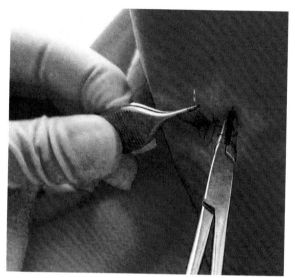

Fig. 13.3 Grasp the short end with the needle holder.

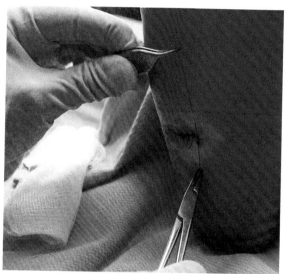

Fig. 13.4 Tie the knot.

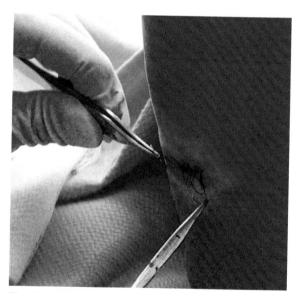

Fig. 13.5 Reverse throw.

Section 3

Closures and procedures

Circular Incisions as a Guide for Optimal Esthetic Removal

Rationale:

- The relaxed skin tension lines (RSTLs) in certain anatomic locations may be difficult to discern.
- The cutaneous lower lip is a good example.
- RSTLs in younger people are also more difficult to locate, but this can be aided by having the patient pucker, smile, grimace or frown.
- Pinching the skin in various directions also helps.
- Hence, the orientation for a traditional excision may involve some guesswork.
- Excising small lesions as a circle prior to designing the ellipse may circumvent this problem.

Technique:

- The lesion of concern is excised with appropriate margins in the shape of a circle (*Fig. 14.1*).
- After undermining, the defect often assumes an oval configuration, indicating the appropriate direction for scar orientation (*Fig. 14.2*).
- Additionally, in neutral areas, such as the skin of the cutaneous lower lip, the skin surrounding the defect can be pinched to best determine the orientation of the relaxed skin tension lines.
- The defect is then converted to a full elliptical excision by drawing the remainder out along the now exposed appropriate axis and closure completed (*Figs 14.3 and 14.4*).
- Or alternatively, the central stitches are placed and the dog-ears at both apices are removed by standard equal-side triangulation of the defect or 'hockey stick' technique.
- Both approaches accomplish the same end.

Advantages:

- This technique offers the advantage of more exact orientation of the final scar within the relaxed skin tension lines.
- In addition, it is a tissue-sparing technique, as often a smaller excision can be done (depending on skin thickness and elasticity) then if it had been planned in a traditional 3:1 ratio.

Caveats:

- This technique requires that the excision be done as two sequential incisions, resulting in a slightly longer operating time.
- If being done for excision of a malignancy, the location of the standing tissue cone removals should be noted and each specimen sent individually to pathology just in case the margin was positive on the initial circular excision at their location.

References:

Salasche SL, Bernstein G, Senkarik M, eds. Surgical anatomy of the skin. Norwalk, Conn: Appleton & Lange; 1988:33–35.

Stegman SJ. Guidelines for the placement of elective incisions. Dermatol Allerg 1980; 3:43–52.

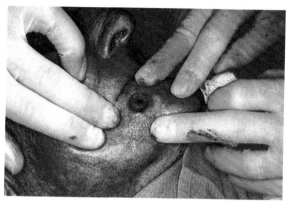

Fig. 14.1 Defect of a cutaneous lower lip lesion excised in the shape of a circle. (From Salasche SL, Bernstein G, Senkarik M, eds. Surgical anatomy of the skin. Norwalk: Appleton & Lange; 1988.)

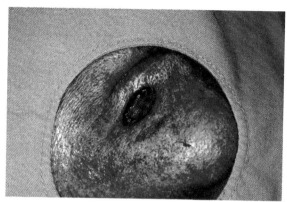

Fig. 14.2 After undermining, the defect assumed an oval shape, better defining the relaxed skin tension lines. (From Salasche SL, Bernstein G, Senkarik M, eds. Surgical anatomy of the skin. Norwalk: Appleton & Lange; 1988.)

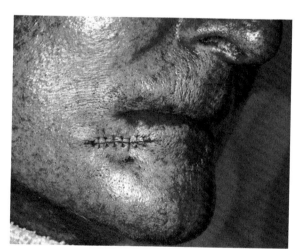

Fig. 14.3 Closure completed. (From Salasche SL, Bernstein G, Senkarik M, eds. Surgical anatomy of the skin. Norwalk: Appleton & Lange; 1988.)

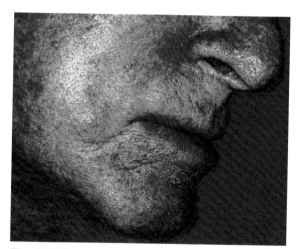

Fig. 14.4 Long-term follow-up. (From Salasche SL, Bernstein G, Senkarik M, eds. Surgical anatomy of the skin. Norwalk: Appleton & Lange; 1988.)

The Crescentic Ellipse for Curving Relaxed Skin Tension Lines

 Rationale:
- Relaxed skin tension lines (RSTLs) of the face are often curved.
- Traditional lenticular ellipses are centered on a straight line.
- If the excisional shape is not modified to accommodate the arc of the RSTLs, a suboptimal esthetic outcome may result.
- Where C-shaped RSTLs exist, the crescentic ellipse variation is beneficial (*Figs 15.1, 15.2, 15.3 and 15.4*).

 Technique:
- Mark the necessary margins around the lesion to be excised.
- The excision should be designed to follow the RSTLs.
- Draw the planned crescentic excision with a convex shape on the convex side of the RSTL and a straight or minimally concave shape on the concave side of the RSTL (*Fig. 15.5*).
- Carry out the excision and proceed with the repair, closing the longer convex side of the defect to the shorter straight or partially concave side using the rule of halves (*Figs 15.6, 15.7 and 15.8*).

 Advantages:
- A crescentic excision allows a more precise placement of the surgical scar within RSTLs with the highest degree of scar camouflage.
- This modified elliptical excision is very helpful on certain areas such as the upper lateral face (over the malar eminence) and along the melolabial fold.

 Caveat:
- This modification is technically more demanding than simple excision and requires solid technical surgical fundamentals to assure the desired result.

 References:
Bennett RG, ed. Basic excisional surgery. In: Fundamentals of cutaneous surgery. St. Louis, Mo: CV Mosby; 1988:434–437.

Odland PB, Kumasaka BH. Fusiform (elliptic) excisions and variations. In: Lask GP, Moy RL, eds. Principles and techniques of cutaneous surgery. New York: McGraw-Hill; 1996:204–205.

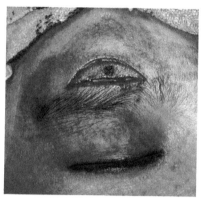

Fig. 15.1 Blue nevus above arched eyebrow.

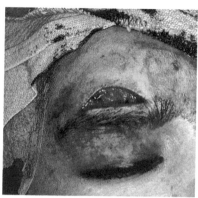

Fig. 15.2 Crescent excised. Convex side arched upward.

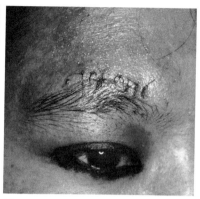

Fig. 15.3 Closed by rule of halves.

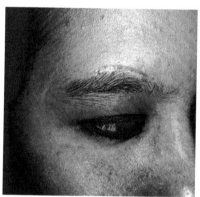

Fig. 15.4 Short-term healing with arch preserved.

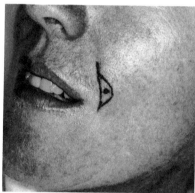

Fig. 15.5 Crescentic excision design on cheek.

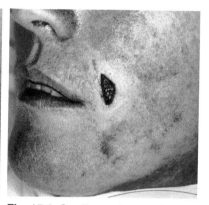

Fig. 15.6 Curvilinear closure of defect: initial stitch using rule of halves.

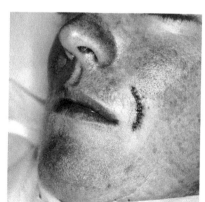

Fig. 15.7 Second and third set of stitches.

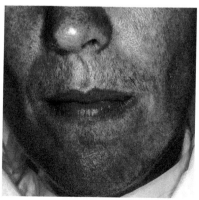

Fig. 15.8 Curvilinear surface closure line within relaxed skin tension lines.

Rationale:

- Certain large or square/rectangular lesions, if totally excised in a single session, would result in spread scars, scars that are longer than necessary or wounds that are closed under excessive tension.
- Because the skin has the ability to stretch, serial or staged excisions may alleviate all these problems.
- Serial excision is particularly amenable to intermediate-sized congenital nevi that are presenting more of a cosmetic problem than a danger of melanoma (*Fig. 16.1*).

Technique:

- A surgical plan is devised to include the anticipated requisite number of excisions.
- This usually involves two or three serial procedures at about 3-month intervals.
- The initial excision should encompass a central portion of the lesion, but should not extend beyond the borders of the lesion (*Fig. 16.2*).
- The width should allow for removal of significant tissue, but should close under little tension (*Fig. 16.3*).
- After the appropriate interval of time, the second (or subsequent) excisions are performed.
- This should include the original scar and the remainder or portions of the residual lesion (*Fig. 16.4*).
- The final result should encompass the entire lesion, and minimally exceed the original length of it (*Fig. 16.5*).
- The final result is often quite acceptable (*Fig. 16.6*).

Caveats:

- There is a certain limit the skin can stretch; if exceeded, a spread scar will result.
- Remove as much of the original lesion as possible with each session.

Reference:

Bennett RG. Fundamentals of cutaneous surgery. St. Louis: CV Mosby; 1988:436–438.

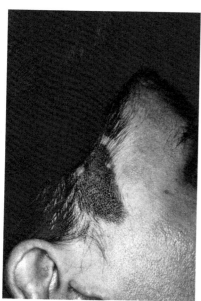

Fig. 16.1 Congenital nevus of temple at hairline.

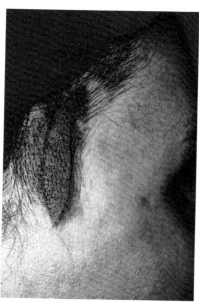

Fig. 16.2 Proposed initial excision.

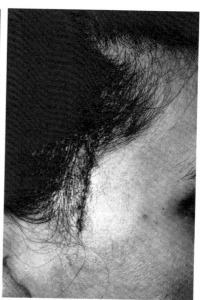

Fig. 16.3 Initial excision complete.

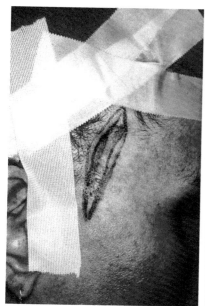

Fig. 16.4 Subsequent excision plan several months later.

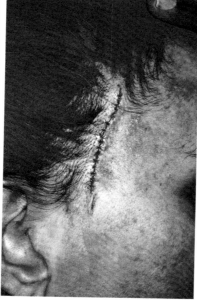

Fig. 16.5 Excision complete: to include the entire residual lesion and scar.

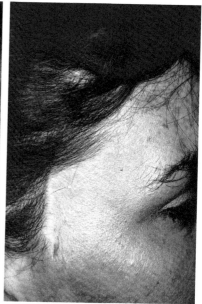

Fig. 16.6 Final result.

Rationale:

- Relaxed skin tension lines (RSTLs) are often curved and/or have a change in contour.
- Therefore, they exist not in a two-dimensional, but in a three-dimensional plane.
- A simple linear closure done over a convex surface such as an arm or leg or the malar eminence of the face may result in a depressed scar as the scar matures and contracts.
- A similar closure done over a concave surface may result in an elevated or band-like scar.
- An S-plasty excision utilizes a longer initial incision line which accommodates for the scar shortening that occurs with scar maturation.
- The two opposing rotation flaps that constitute an S-plasty draw on a larger reservoir so that as scar maturation and shortening occurs, normal contours are re-established.

Technique:

- The appropriate margins are drawn around the lesion to be excised (Figs 17.1 and 17.2).
- Each half of the 'S' is drawn as half of a crescentic ellipse with one the reverse image of the other.
- Whenever possible, the long axis of the ellipse should be in a relaxed skin tension line (Fig. 17.3).
- After excision and undermining, the wound edges are rotated in opposite directions and then advanced toward one another with the first suture placed along the midpoint of each side (Fig. 17.4).

- This essentially accomplishes three separate closures with different tension vectors of closure (Fig. 17.4).
- Closure then follows by the rule of halves (Figs 17.5 and 17.6).

Advantages:

- An S-shaped excision respects the three-dimensional anatomic contours of the surgical field.
- Closures that cross from convex to concave surfaces are accommodated by three separate tension vectors of closure.
- Irregularities such as scar banding over concave areas or scar depression over convex areas, which might cause functional or esthetic compromise, are less likely to occur.

Caveats:

- Because of the 'S' configuration one or both of the tips of the S-plasty will, by necessity, cross the RSTLs.
- The design as well as the performance of an S-plasty is more technically demanding than a simple excision.

References:

Arpey CJ, Whitaker DC, O'Donnell MJ, eds. Excisional and elliptical–fusiform variations. In: Cutaneous surgery – illustrated and practical approach. New York: McGraw-Hill; 1997:62–63.

Odland PB, Kumasaka BH. Fusiform (elliptic) excisions and variations. In: Lask GP, Moy RL, eds. Principles and techniques of cutaneous surgery. New York: McGraw-Hill; 1996:205–207.

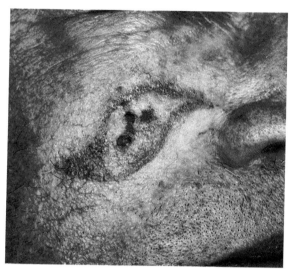

Fig. 17.1 S-plasty markings with its long axis centered on the RSTLs. (From Salasche SJ, Bernstein G, Senkarik M. Surgical anatomy of the skin. Norwalk, Appelton & Lange, 1988.)

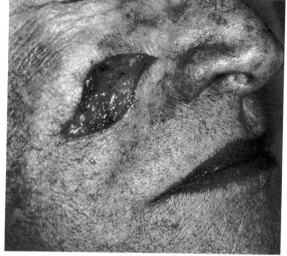

Fig. 17.2 Defect following excision. (From Salasche SJ, Bernstein G, Senkarik M. Surgical anatomy of the skin. Norwalk, Appelton & Lange, 1988.)

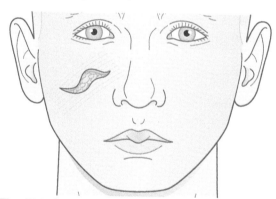

Fig. 17.3 S-plasty centered on the long axis. Note the greater tip-to-tip distance for the S-plasty versus a traditional ellipse.

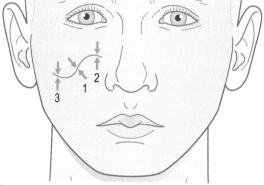

Fig. 17.4 The center portion is closed first. The divided-off two segments are then initially closed at the midpoint. There are three separate tension vectors.

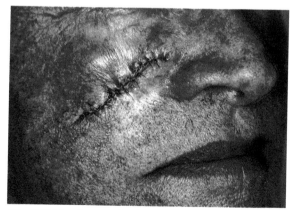

Fig. 17.5 Lesion repaired.

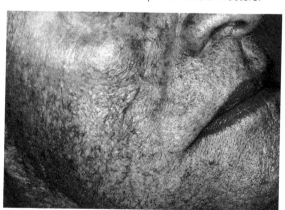

Fig. 17.6 After suture removal.

Rationale:

- Second-intention healing may be the treatment of choice for certain defects or it may be chosen because of extenuating circumstances (e.g. the patient is a smoker) (*Fig. 18.1*).
- Occasionally, and for no known reason, exuberant granulation tissue ('proud flesh') develops.
- This hypergranulation appears as a beefy red, spongy mat above the level of the surrounding skin (*Fig. 18.2*).
- It can delay or inhibit healing by preventing inward migration and final coverage by the epidermis.

Technique:

- Standard technique is to curette the excessive granulation flush with the surrounding skin (*Fig. 18.3*).
- This may be a bit painful, usually doesn't require anesthesia, and may cause bleeding.
- An alternative technique is to firmly apply a silver nitrate applicator stick (75% $AgNO_3$) (*Fig. 18.4*).
- This turns the area white initially, but then it turns gray.
- The tissue becomes necrotic and sloughs after about 1–2 weeks (depending on size and thickness of the exuberant granulation tissue).
- At this point, epithelialization usually progresses until healing is complete (*Figs 18.5 and 18.6*).
- The silver nitrate may need to reapplied if persistent proud flesh is noted.

Advantages:

- Easy to apply.
- No anesthesia is required and silver nitrate is also an anticoagulant.
- Can be reapplied if necessary.

Caveat:

- Can leave a dermal tattoo, especially if area is large.

Reference:

Bennett RC. Fundamentals of cutaneous surgery. St. Louis: CV Mosby; 1988:501.

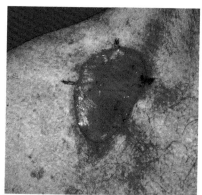

Fig. 18.1 Initial detect.

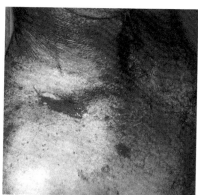

Fig. 18.2 Second-intention healing wound with 'proud flesh.'

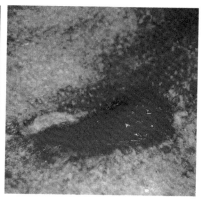

Fig. 18.3 Close-up showing raised granulations and stagnant epidermis.

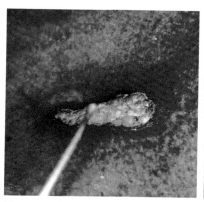

Fig. 18.4 Silver nitrate application.

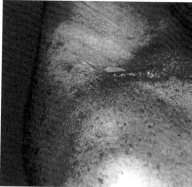

Fig. 18.5 Almost healed.

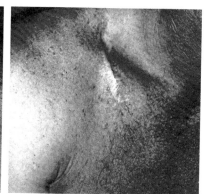

Fig. 18.6 Healed wound.

Hydrodissection (Hydroplaning) with Anesthetic Fluid

 Rationale:
- Injecting a bolus of anesthetic fluid into the skin imparts volume-related properties other than impairing nerve conduction.
- Depending on the depth within the skin and the volume of fluid injected, these properties include distending the skin to make it less mobile, thicker and more rigid.
- These changes can be used to advantage in various dermatologic procedures.
- These include curettage and desiccation, obtaining a very thin disc of tissue for frozen section and for separating the overlying skin from the perichondrium or periosteum.
- As demonstrated here, separating the overlying skin from the perichondrium or periosteum is helpful in predetermining if a tumor involves the underlying cartilage or bone.

 Technique:
- If the intent is to separate the plane above the perichondrium or periosteum, the needle is inserted into the plane just above the membrane and fluid is slowly injected (*Figs 19.1 and 19.2*).
- The supraperichondrial space is distended and expanded (*Fig. 19.3*).
- If the plane is free of tumor, it would usually hydrodissect quite easily under the tumor (*Fig. 19.4*).
- The surgeon can use curved, blunt-ended tissue scissors to dissect out the tumor within this plane (*Figs 19.5 and 19.6*).
- Surgical dissection should be carried out soon after hydrodissection is done as fluid will dissipate within a short time.

 Advantages:
- May provide information about depth of invasion of tumors at the bone or cartilage level.
- Facilitates dissection of the tumor.
- May preserve cartilage.
- Allow for healing by graft or second intention if perichondrium is preserved.

 Caveat:
- Needle must be placed at appropriate level in skin for intended goal.

 Reference:
Salasche SJ, Giancola JM, Trookman NS. Hydro-expansion with anesthetic fluid. J Am Acad Dermatol 1995; 33:510–512.

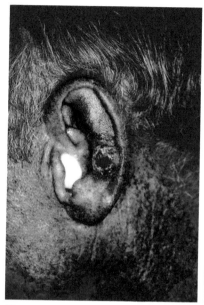

Fig. 19.1 KA-like squamous cell carcinoma of the ear.

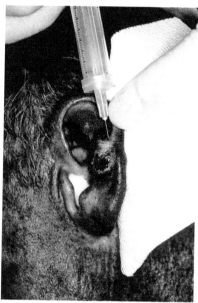

Fig. 19.2 Needle inserted into supraperichondrial plane. (From Salasche SJ, Giancola JM, Trookman NS. Hydro-expansion with anesthetic fluid. J Am Acad Dermatol 1995; 33:510–512.)

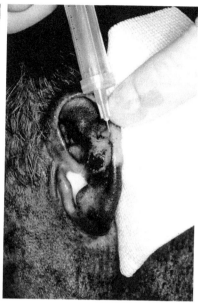

Fig. 19.3 Hydroplaning initiated. (From Salasche SJ, Giancola JM, Trookman NS. Hydro-expansion with anesthetic fluid. J Am Acad Dermatol 1995; 33:510–512.)

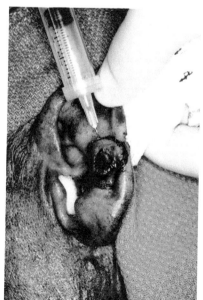

Fig. 19.4 Entire tumor hydrodissected.

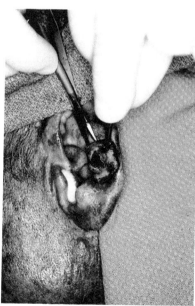

Fig. 19.5 Excision above perichondrium. (From Salasche SJ, Giancola JM, Trookman NS. Hydro-expansion with anesthetic fluid. J Am Acad Dermatol 1995; 33:510–512.)

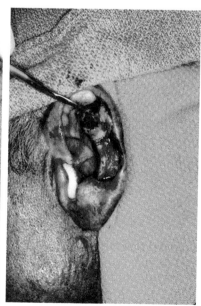

Fig. 19.6 Tumor removed with perichondrium intact.

Rationale:

- Bare cartilage on the ear devoid of its covering perichondrium will not support a skin graft or heal by second-intention healing.
- There has to be a covering of tissue capable of propagating granulation tissue.
- Large denuded defects would be prone to necrosis if second-intention healing were attempted and, similarly, grafts would fail.
- Tissue rearrangements (flaps) are a possible solution as they bring their own blood supply; however, there may not be much available skin to cover large ear defects.
- The technique below is geared to generating granulation tissue from the perichondrium on the other side of the cartilage under the defect.
- This granulation tissue will fill the punch defect, migrate out over the bare cartilage and bridge the gap between punches until the entire defect is covered.

 Technique:

- The tissue on the reverse side of the defect is anesthetized with local infiltration of lidocaine with epinephrine.
- Under sterile conditions, 4 mm punch biopsies are used to remove, in a cookie cutter manner, cores of cartilage down to the perichondrium on the opposite side of the defect (Figs 20.1 and 20.2).
- Cutting through the cartilage itself is not painful and is quite easy to accomplish with gentle, twisting, downward pressure on the punch.
- There is some resistance when the perichondrium is reached, which should signal cessation of the cutting pressure.
- The cartilage cores are easily removed with a toothed forceps.

- Sufficient holes are punched to insure sufficient granulation tissue is generated as well as maintaining the integrity of the ear structure (Fig. 20.3).
- Leaving at least 4 mm in all directions around the punch site suffices.
- Pressure with sterile gauze alone is used to attain hemostasis.
- The wound is dressed with antibiotic ointment-impregnated gauze or antibiotic and a non-stick dressing pad, which is changed on a daily basis.
- After several days, granulation tissue appears in each of the 'planters' and subsequently fills the punch holes and spread out over the bare cartilage until it meets up with neighboring outgrowths and the entire surface is covered (Figs 20.4 and 20.5).
- Either a delayed split- or full-thickness skin graft is placed or the wound is allowed to continue on to heal completely by second intention.
- Complete epithelialization of the surface completes this process (Fig. 20.6).

 Caveats:

- Opposite side of cartilage must be anesthetized.
- Don't push too hard on the punch, to avoid injuring perichondrium on opposite side.
- During healing, the wound bed must be continuously hydrated to avoid desiccation.

 References:

Albom MJ. Surgical gems. J Derm Surg Oncol 1975; 1:60.

Salasche SJ, Winton GB, Adnot A. Surgical pearls. Dermatol Clin 1989; 7:75–110.

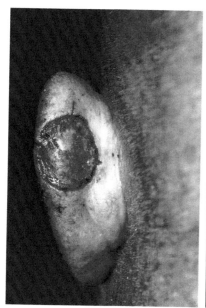

Fig. 20.1 Post tumor-removal defect of posterior ear; devoid of perichondrium.

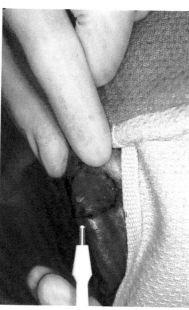

Fig. 20.2 Cores of cartilage removed with 4 mm punch biopsy.

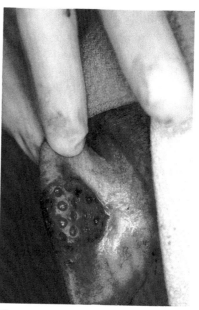

Fig. 20.3 Sufficient cores removed to retain integrity of cartilage.

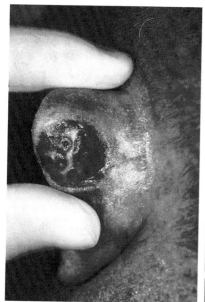

Fig. 20.4 Two weeks: granulation tissue migrating across bare cartilage.

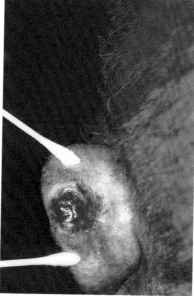

Fig. 20.5 Three weeks: granulation bridges wound and early inward advance of epithelial sheet.

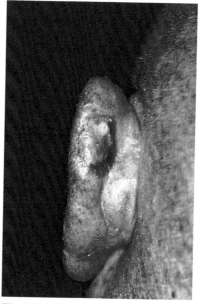

Fig. 20.6 Five weeks: wound completely covered.

A User-Friendly Surgical Dressing

Rationale:
- Patients are often incapable or reluctant to participate in their own dressing changes.
- Enlisting help from family, friends or visiting nurse may be inconvenient and may incur extra expense.
- Incorrect performance of dressing changes and wound care may cause inadvertent harm.
- A dressing that remains untouched and intact from the postsurgical period until suture removal is beneficial.
- The dressing should perform all the usual functions of initial immobilization of the wound, protect the suture line and provide a hydrated environment for wound healing.

Technique:
- The only materials required are flesh-toned Micropore paper tape (3M), liquid adhesive Mastisol ampules (Ferndale Laboratories) and an antibiotic ointment of choice.
- The 'inner' portion of the dressing is fashioned from a double- or triple-layer strip of tape (Fig. 21.1).
- After surgery is completed, the suture line is coated with a fine layer of the petrolatum-based ointment.
- The area surrounding the ointment is then coated with a film of the Mastisol adhesive (either directly from the ampule applicator or by cotton-tipped applicator from the plastic bottle container) (Fig. 21.2).
- After the liquid adhesive has dried to a 'tacky' state after about 15–30 seconds (depending on the thickness of application), the trimmed multilayered inner dressing is placed sticky side down over the suture line (Fig. 21.3).
- The portion of tape actually applied to the wound is cut off below the attachment to the wooden or metal shelf used to prepare the multilayered strip (Fig. 21.1).
- This inner dressing covers both the areas coated with ointment and the surrounding area coated with the adhesive.

- Then the area around the inner dressing is again painted with liquid adhesive and an 'outer' compressive dressing is fashioned (Fig. 21.4).
- This may consist of folded gauze pads or dental rolls which are placed over the inner dressing.
- The outer dressing is secured with sufficient tape strips, which are arranged to run in the opposite direction from the inner dressing (Figs 21.5 and 21.6).
- Patients may remove the outer compressive dressing after 24 hours.
- They are instructed to start the removal by loosening the tape from either side up toward the middle.
- The inner dressing stays intact until suture removal (Figs 21.7 and 21.8).
- It is usually esthetically acceptable and trouble-free.
- There may be some discoloration from the antibiotic ointment.

Advantages:
- Patients do not have to look at their wound.
- They do not have to participate in wound care.
- There are no extra expenses for dressing materials.

Caveats:
- If bleeding or pain/tenderness occurs, patient should be instructed to communicate with doctor.
- Since repair is not visible, early signs of infection may be covered up.
- In the event the inner dressing comes off, written instructions for wound care must be provided when the patient leaves the office.

Reference:
Fewkes JL, Salasche SJ. Surgical pearl: a user-friendly dressing. J Am Acad Dermatol 1993; 29:633–635.

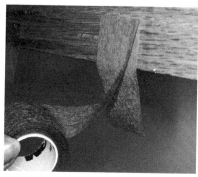

Fig. 21.1 Multilayered 'inner' dressing strip being prepared. Only portion below attachment to wood is placed on patient. (From Fewkes JL, Salasche SJ. Surgical pearl: a user-friendly dressing. J Am Acad Dermatol 1993; 29:633–635.)

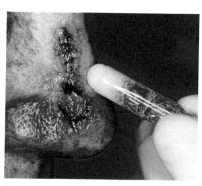

Fig. 21.2 Liquid adhesive applied to area around suture line. (From Fewkes JL, Salasche SJ. Surgical pearl: a user-friendly dressing. J Am Acad Dermatol 1993; 29:633–635.)

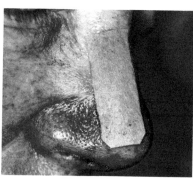

Fig. 21.3 Trimmed 'inner' dressing in place. (From Fewkes JL, Salasche SJ. Surgical pearl: a user-friendly dressing. J Am Acad Dermatol 1993; 29:633–635.)

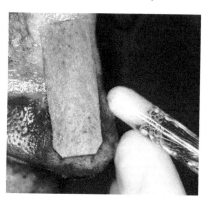

Fig. 21.4 Liquid adhesive placed around inner dressing.

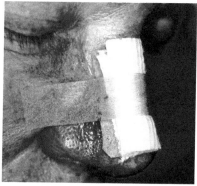

Fig. 21.5 Outer dressing secured. (From Fewkes JL, Salasche SJ. Surgical pearl: a user-friendly dressing. J Am Acad Dermatol 1993; 29:633–635.)

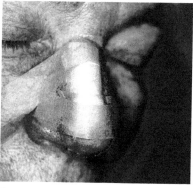

Fig. 21.6 Outer dressing: tape runs opposite to inner dressing.

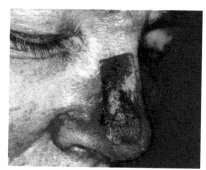

Fig. 21.7 Inner dressing on 5th postoperative day. (From Fewkes JL, Salasche SJ. Surgical pearl: a user-friendly dressing. J Am Acad Dermatol 1993; 29:633–635.)

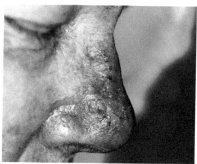

Fig. 21.8 Inner dressing removed prior to suture removal on 5th day. (From Fewkes JL, Salasche SJ. Surgical pearl: a user-friendly dressing. J Am Acad Dermatol 1993; 29:633–635.)

Minimizing the Dog-Ear: Good Use of Fingers and String

Rationale:

- Sometimes even well-planned elliptical closures don't line up as designed.
- This can be due to overly elastic skin wherein the nicely designed ellipse converts to a circle.
- Or if the skin is thick or elastotic, the apical angles have to be even more acute than anticipated.
- Sometimes, if the design was drawn when the patient was not in rest position, the tension lines may have been misread.
- Undermining and freeing up the surrounding skin only exaggerates the situation.
- Two simple maneuvers can alleviate the problem.

Technique:

- An example is shown of an excisional biopsy of a pigmented lesion on the abdomen of a 19-year-old young lady (*Fig. 22.1*).
- As the ellipse is performed, the surrounding elastic skin retracts in all directions and a wider, more oval defect results (*Fig. 22.2*).
- Simply stretching the skin outward and parallel to the long axis of the defect realigns the elliptical design (*Fig. 22.3*).
- This works best if the long axis is designed to parallel the relaxed skin tension lines (RSTLs).
- This can be further refined by placing the first side of the buried vertical mattress suture and tugging it toward the opposite side to find the best 'fit' that eliminates any potential dog-ear (*Fig. 22.4*).
- Even better is to combine both maneuvers (*Fig. 22.5*).
- After this suture is tied, the procedure is continued with additional buried sutures until the wound is secured without dog-ears and ready for the final surface stitches (*Fig. 22.6*).

Advantage:

- By stretching the skin parallel to the RSTL while using a guiding suture, the wound can be accurately closed and dog-ears eliminated.

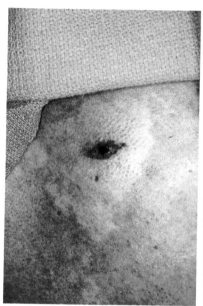

Fig. 22.1 Classic elliptical design.

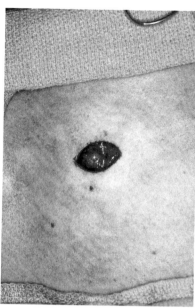

Fig. 22.2 Forms oval defect after excision.

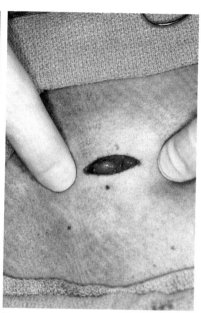

Fig. 22.3 Stretching the skin realigns ellipse.

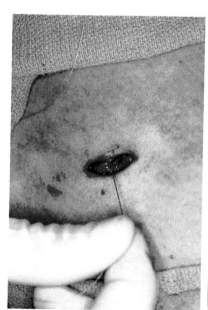

Fig. 22.4 Using half-buried stitch to orient closure.

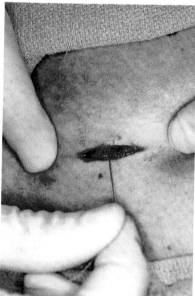

Fig. 22.5 Combining both techniques to bisect wound.

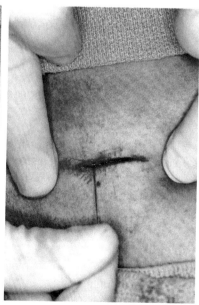

Fig. 22.6 Second buried stitch refines any potential dog-ear.

Rationale:

- The standard 4.0 mm punch biopsy is a routine dermatologic procedure.
- The punch site can be left to heal by second intention or it can be stitched primarily.
- Standard procedure for attempting to achieve a linear closure of the circular defect is to:
- Stretch the skin opposite the skin lines before the punch is executed, and
- Use a single interrupted or vertical mattress suture to direct the closure parallel to the prevailing relaxed skin tension lines (RSTLs).
- Despite this, dog-ears may develop in thick or elastotic skin.
- A couple of refinements in technique may further alleviate dog-ear formation.
- These include the use of two interrupted stitches and stretching the skin parallel to the RSTL to define the long axis of closure.

Technique:

- The RSTLs of the region are clearly defined.
- Just before inserting the punch biopsy, the skin is firmly stretched perpendicular (opposite) to the RSTL with the thumb and index finger of the surgeon's non-dominant hand (Fig. 23.1).
- After the punch biopsy tissue is snipped and extracted at its base and tension is released, the biopsy site defect usually assumes an oval configuration parallel to the RSTL (Fig. 23.2).
- The long axis of the oval defines the direction of closure.
- Suture placement is aided by gently stretching the skin with the thumb and index of the surgeon's non-dominant hand, but this time at the opposite ends of the long axis of closure (i.e. parallel to the RSTL) (Fig. 23.3).
- This maneuver exaggerates the linear nature of the defect and allows placement of each stitch about one-third from each now more clearly defined 'apex' (Fig. 23.4).
- The defect is then closed with two simple interrupted stitches (Fig. 23.4).

Advantages:

- Punch biopsies can be cosmetically pleasing as well as quick, simple and functional.
- Depending on thickness and elasticity of the skin, a nearly linear closure can be attained without bulges at each end.
- Takes longer than the routine technique, but worth it, especially on the face and neck.

Reference:

Olbricht S. Biopsy techniques and basic excisions. In: Bolognia J, Jorizzo J, Rapini R, eds. Dermatology. London: Mosby; 2003:2269–2286.

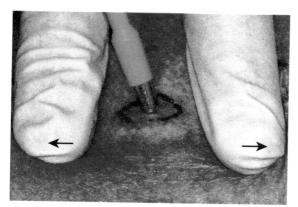

Fig. 23.1 Skin stretched in the opposite direction to RSTL.

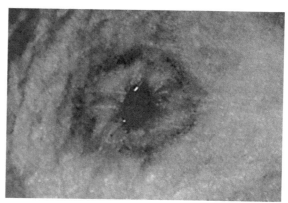

Fig. 23.2 Oval configuration after biopsy removed.

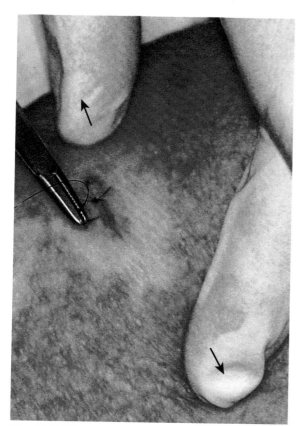

Fig. 23.3 Ellipse accentuated by stretching parallel to long axis.

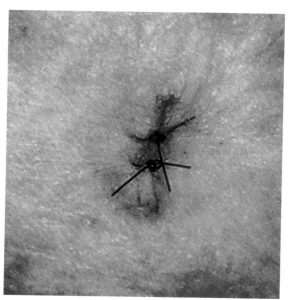

Fig. 23.4 Defect closed with two stitches.

Rationale:

- The punch biopsy is a standard method of obtaining tissue for histologic diagnosis of diseases of the skin.
- Routinely, the entire specimen is transferred to the laboratory in formalin for processing into standard histopathology slides.
- Occasionally, the differential diagnosis dictates that tissue be obtained for other studies that would be adversely affected by formalin fixation.
- These include tissue culture for deep fungi, atypical mycobacteria or bacteria.
- Similarly, tissue destined for immunofluorescence studies or electron microscopy requires freezing or special fixation.
- Therefore, in these situations, the punch specimen needs to be divided.
- Division is accomplished by scalpel or razor blade, but may prove cumbersome as the small specimen is difficult to stabilize.
- Rough handling of the tissue may cause crush injury or uneven sections.
- The following technique simplifies the process.

Technique:

- The skin is routinely prepped and anesthetized.
- The punch is inserted into the skin, but only to the depth of the papillary dermis and is then withdrawn (*Figs 24.1 and 24.2*).
- Using a #11 blade, the tissue is bisected to a depth that reaches down 3–4 mm into the reticular dermis (*Fig. 24.3*).
- The punch is then reintroduced and is rotated and advanced to complete the biopsy into the subcutaneous fat (*Fig. 24.4*).
- The partially bisected specimen is removed with the aid of a scissors and untoothed forceps (*Fig. 24.5*).
- The specimen is placed on a tongue depressor or gauze (*Fig. 24.6*).
- Bisection is completed with a scalpel or razor blade (*Figs 24.7 and 24.8*).

Advantages:

- This technique simplifies the bisection procedure by stabilizing the tissue while still tethered in the skin.
- Crush injury is avoided.
- Some make the bisecting cut all the way into the subcutaneous fat, but the fully cut tissue may be difficult to remove.

Reference:

Inman VD, Pariser RJ. Biopsy technique pearl: obtaining an optimal split punch-biopsy specimen. J Am Acad Dermatol 2003; 48:273–274.

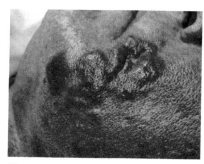

Fig. 24.1 Punch is introduced just into skin suspected of being an infectious granuloma.

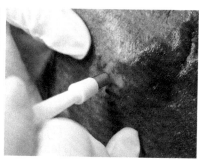

Fig. 24.2 Surface is scored down to level of papillary dermis and first capillary bleeding.

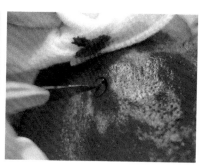

Fig. 24.3 Appearance (cross-bun) after partial bisection.

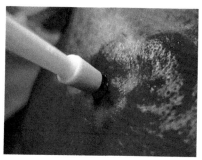

Fig. 24.4 Punch is reintroduced and advanced to level of subcutaneous fat.

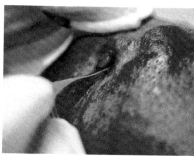

Fig. 24.5 Specimen is removed.

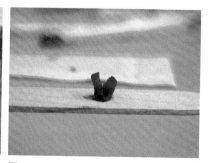

Fig. 24.6 Partially bisected specimen on wooden tongue depressor.

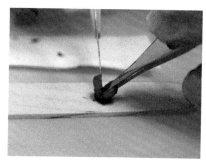

Fig. 24.7 Tissue divided.

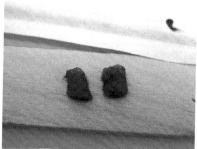

Fig. 24.8 Two pieces.

Saucerization Biopsy

 Rationale:

- Many lesions require biopsy to obtain tissue for histologic examination.
- The shave, punch, incision/excision biopsy hierarchy suffices for most situations.
- However, some lesions can be adequately examined with saucerized excision.
- Small, thin, pigmented lesions on the trunk or extremities that are not highly suspicious for melanoma, but require histologic examination, fall into this portion of the spectrum.
- Examples are some solar lentigines or dysplastic nevi.
- The technique is predicated on removing the entire lesion and small portions of peripheral and deep normal-appearing tissue.

 Technique:

- The surgical site is prepped and anesthetized.
- The intended margin (1–2 mm) of the biopsy is marked with a surgical marker, or preferably, by incising just into the papillary dermis circumferentially around the lesion (Fig. 25.1).
- This will provide an indelible guide for the extent of the cutting.
- Next, another bolus of anesthetic fluid is injected just under the lesion to help raise it up and also provide a stiff, firm field upon which to work.
- At a safe distance, the operator uses the thumb and index finger of his non-dominant hand to push the surrounding tissue inward under the lesion, effectively also elevating it (Figs 25.2 and 25.3).
- Using a #15 or #10 scalpel held parallel to the skin, and using a sawing motion along the surface markings, the tumor is removed to the required depth (Figs 25.3 and 25.4).
- Alternatively, a razor blade can be used.
- The depth is usually to the lower reticular dermis or upper subcutaneous fat.
- The entire specimen is freed and the base and perimeter checked for residual pigment (Fig. 25.5).
- Hemostasis is attained with aluminum chloride (Fig. 25.6).
- Wound care is daily cleansing, application of a petrolatum-based ointment and a non-adherent dressing.

 Advantages:

- When cases are appropriately selected, full excision and suturing is avoided.
- In the areas selected (back, shoulders, upper arms) the final outcome of the scarring is often comparable to excision and suturing, especially if multiple lesions are removed over time.
- Costs are lower.
- The saucerization is essentially a complete excision of the lesion with a rim of clinically normal tissue.
- It should provide all the histologic data, as with formal excision.

 Caveat:

- Insure the entire lesion is removed.

Reference:

Orengo I, Katta R, Rosen T. Techniques in the removal of skin lesions. Otolaryngol Clin N Am 2002; 34:153–170.

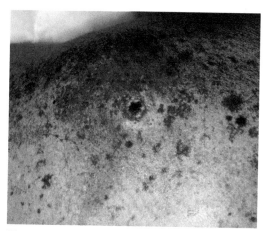

Fig. 25.1 Thin dysplastic nevus on upper back with proposed excision.

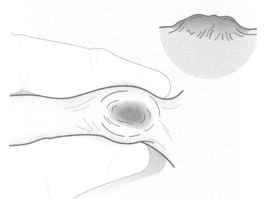

Fig. 25.2 Skin bunched under lesion to elevate and stabilize.

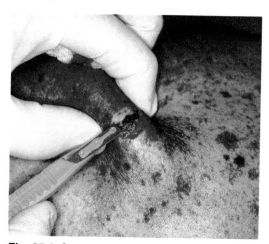

Fig. 25.3 Saucerization underway.

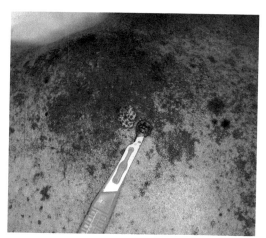

Fig. 25.4 Complete removal of lesion with rim of normal tissue.

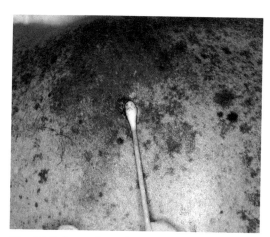

Fig. 25.5 Base clear of pigment. Depth at deep reticular dermis interface with subcutaneous fat.

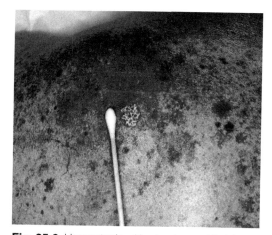

Fig. 25.6 Hemostasis with aluminum chloride.

TIP 26

'Off-set Bias Suturing' to Favorably Alter the Tension Vector of Closure

Rationale:

- As noted, unfavorable tension vectors (TVs) can distort free margins and lead to functional problems and/or cosmetic asymmetries.
- There are several methods of altering the tension vector of closure.
- Flaps (tissue rearrangements) can be used when side-to-side closure would result in a poor tension vector.
- Full-thickness grafts prevent wound contraction and may be used as alternatives to second-intention healing and other closures for this purpose.
- As noted in Tip 37, suspension (pexing or anchoring) sutures into the periosteum can alter tension vectors.
- Yet another maneuver, 'off-set bias suturing', can be used to favorably shift the tension vector.

Technique:

- When pre-suture testing or initial closure identifies an unfavorable side-to-side TV, an alternative method should be considered (*Figs 26.1–26.4*).
- Buried sutures are placed to shift the direction of closure.
- These sutures often suffice to accomplish the reoriented TV.
- Once this is accomplished, the remaining surface sutures are placed (*Figs 26.2 and 26.5*).
- The final outcome should reflect the corrected TV direction (*Fig. 26.6*).

Advantage:

- This is a rather simple solution that uses the original plan for a primary closure.

Caveats:

- Inherent to using offset bias-suturing is shifting of the tissue on each side of the wound, so that dog-ears or more extensive dog-ears are created at each end.
- These should be excised as part of the final closure to insure the intended result.

References:

Salasche SJ. Complications of excisional surgery. In: Theirs BH, Lange BH, Lange PG, Jnr (eds) Yearbook of Dermatology and Dermatologic Surgery, Mosby, St. Louis, 2002.

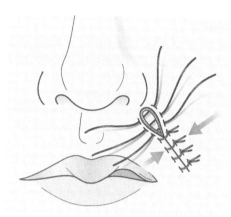

Fig. 26.1 Closure of melolabial fold defect elevates corner of mouth.

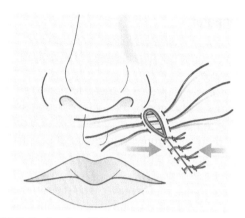

Fig. 26.2 Redirecting TV horizontally corrects problem.

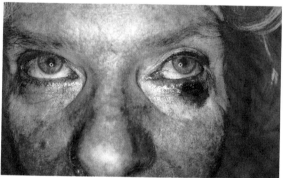

Fig. 26.3 Defect of lower lid near lid margin. (From Theirs BH, Lange BH, Lange PG, Jnr (eds) Yearbook of Dermatology and Dermatologic Surgery, Mosby, St. Louis, 2002.)

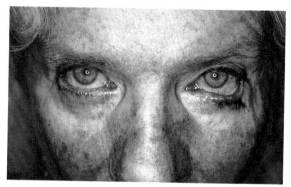

Fig. 26.4 Proposed closure would cause ectropion. (From Theirs BH, Lange BH, Lange PG, Jnr (eds) Yearbook of Dermatology and Dermatologic Surgery, Mosby, St. Louis, 2002.)

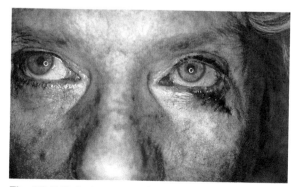

Fig. 26.5 Defect re-sutured with more favorable horizontal tension vector. (From Theirs BH, Lange BH, Lange PG, Jnr (eds) Yearbook of Dermatology and Dermatologic Surgery, Mosby, St. Louis, 2002.)

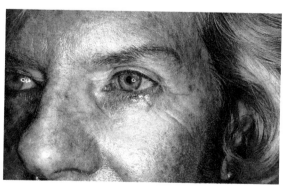

Fig. 26.6 Short-term healing.

Have I Cut the Temporal Nerve or Just Anesthetized It?

 Rationale:

- Deeply invasive basal cell and squamous cell carcinoma occur relatively commonly on the temple.
- Surgical extirpation of these tumors places the temporal branch of the facial nerve at risk.
- The temporal nerve may be projected on the skin on a line running from about 0.5 cm below the tragus to a point 2 cm above the lateral eyebrow (*Fig. 27.1*).
- Cutting this motor nerve, a single ramus in 85% of people, results in permanent paresis of the frontalis muscle with ipsilateral inability to wrinkle the forehead, raise the eyebrow or open the eye widely (*Fig. 27.2*).
- Equally important is the depth at which the nerve courses within skin: at the temple level it is just below the superficial temporalis fascia – superficial muscular aponeurotic system (SMAS) (*Fig. 27.3*).
- The superficial temporalis fascia is contiguous with the galea aponeurotica of the scalp.
- Single or repeated application of local anesthetic (1% lidocaine and epinephrine) during excisional or Mohs micrographic surgery may result in diffusion of anesthetic down to the nerve and cause a profound nerve block for up to 12 hours.
- If, during the course or at the completion of surgery, the patient displays signs of temporal nerve paresis, a quick clue as to whether one has reached sufficient depth within the skin to have injured the nerve is the following.

 Technique:

- If one can still see subcutaneous fat on the floor of the defect, the nerve has not been cut.
- The problem is when there is a white membrane visible at the defect base.
- Under sterile conditions, with a gloved index finger, try to move the tissue back and forth.
- If it rotates and moves easily, it is the superficial temporal fascia, and most likely the nerve, has not been injured (*Fig. 27.4*).
- If the tissue is glistening white and firmly bound down and not responsive to the finger, the temporalis fascia over the temporal muscle has been reached, a muscle of mastication, and more than likely, if the nerve was in this area, it has been cut (*Fig. 27.4*).

 Advantage:

- The main advantage is to be able to tell if you are superficial to the nerve or not prior to the anesthesia wearing off.

 Caveat:

- Tell patients during informed consent discussions that either temporary or permanent nerve-related symptoms may develop during surgery in this area.

 Reference:

Grabski WJ, Salasche SF. Management of temporal nerve injuries. J Dermatol Surg Oncol 1985; 11:145.

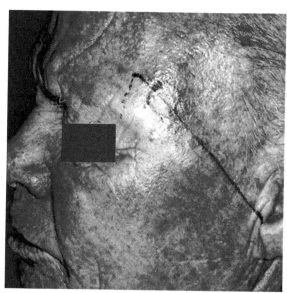

Fig. 27.1 Projected pathway of temporal nerve. (From Grabski WJ, Salasche SF. Management of temporal nerve injuries. J Dermatol Surg Oncol 1985; 11:145.)

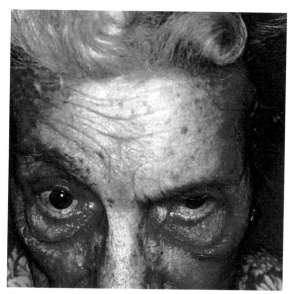

Fig. 27.2 Characteristic facies following severance of temporal nerve. (From Grabski WJ, Salasche SF. Management of temporal nerve injuries. J Dermatol Surg Oncol 1985; 11:145.)

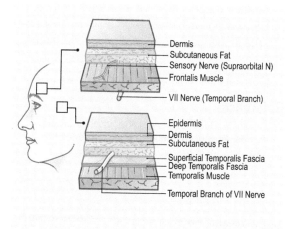

Fig. 27.3 Course of the motor temporal nerve between the SMAS and deep temporal fascia.

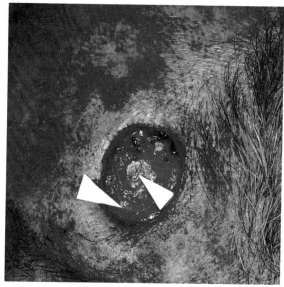

Fig. 27.4 Upper arrow shows superficial temporal fascia (SMAS); lower arrow, the subcutaneous fat.

Rationale:

- Benign epidermal lesions can be treated with several different surgical modalities or even topical agents.
- Common warts are such a condition and variably respond to treatment with liquid nitrogen cryotherapy, cantharidin, podophyllin, or intralesional bleomycin.
- All these may leave scarring or require multiple interventions.
- Recalcitrant common warts on most any location are amenable to electrodesiccation/electrofulguration and curettage.
- Condyloma acuminata, seborrheic keratosis and dermatosis papulosa nigra are also amenable to this treatment.

Technique:

- First, the area is cleansed and then anesthetized with local anesthesia containing epinephrine.
- Light electrodesiccation or electrofulguration of the wart is performed (*Fig. 28.1*).
- The wart is noted to shrink back from the dermis and become smaller.
- Warts are entirely epidermal so care should be taken to not cause damage to the basement membrane or dermis.
- Usually, the surgeon is then able to slide the wart away from the epidermis with lateral motion of the curette (*Figs 28.2, 28.3 and 28.4*).

- Residual bleeding can be stopped with direct pressure, aluminum chloride, or very light spot electrodesiccation.
- Again, care should be taken not to injure sub-basement membrane tissue.
- Palm, sole and even periungual lesions usually respond to this treatment.
- Face lesions should be treated with especial care to prevent scarring or dyspigmentation (*Figs 28.5, 28.6 and 28.7*).
- There is minimal wound care, which consists of daily cleansing, application of petrolatum-based ointment, and a band aid.

Advantages:

- This is a definitive procedure and is often curative, even for previously treated warts.
- It is a single procedure and does not require multiple visits or treatments.

Caveats:

- Treat lightly to minimize hypopigmentation and scarring, especially avoid overtreatment and scarring, especially on the nail unit or face.
- There is potential transmission of HPV or other virus in the electrodesiccation smoke plume.
- A smoke evacuator should be used for this procedure.

Reference:

Robinson JK. Electrosurgery. In: Robinson JK, Arndt KA, et al., eds. Atlas of cutaneous surgery. Philadelphia: WB Saunders; 1996:61–65.

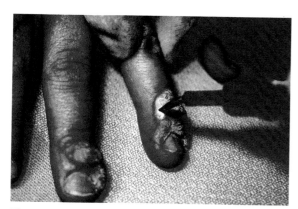

Fig. 28.1 Electrodesiccation of a periungual wart.

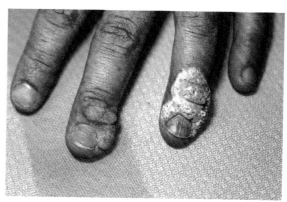

Fig. 28.2 After wart shrinks and retracts, apply firm lateral pressure with curette.

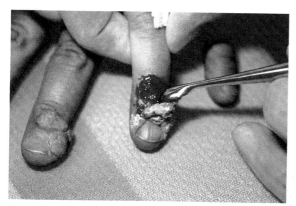

Fig. 28.3 Wart usually slides off or peels away with curette pressure.

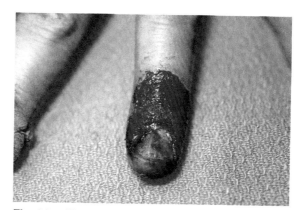

Fig. 28.4 Wart removed cleanly.

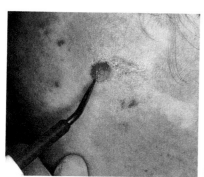

Fig. 28.5 Wart on face: light electrodesiccation.

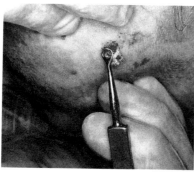

Fig. 28.6 Curettage.

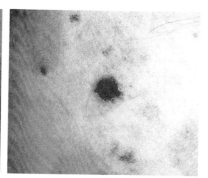

Fig. 28.7 Wart-free after curettage.

Rationale:

- There are a variety of small, benign, space-occupying subepidermal lesions such as epidermoid inclusion cysts, steatocystoma multiplex and lipomas.
- Surgical excision of such lesions is curative and cosmetically acceptable, but in some instances seems excessive for the size and location.
- A simplified approach is to remove the lesion through a small stab or punch wound.

 Technique:

Technique for cyst removal

- After sterile preparation, the skin over, around and under the cyst is locally infiltrated with local anesthesia.
- Care is taken not to inject into the cyst (although not critical).
- With a #11 surgical blade, a small stab wound is made into the cyst cavity.
- Orientation of the blade wound is parallel to the local relaxed skin tension lines (*Fig. 29.1*).
- The wound should be about 3 mm in length to allow entry of a 2 mm curette as well as extrusion of the cyst contents.
- The curette is introduced into the cyst cavity and swept around the entire wall and base (*Fig. 29.2*).
- The curette is removed and the contents expressed by inward digital compression (*Fig. 29.3*).
- A portion of the cyst wall is usually also extruded by this maneuver.
- It can be grasped with a hemostat or forceps and the remainder teased from the wound (*Fig. 29.4*).
- Alternatively, reintroducing the curette will produce the sac.
- Closure can be done with vertical mattress sutures or, if there is little dead space, by an anti-tension strip across the wound and pressure dressing.

Technique for lipoma removal

- Lipomas are benign, encapsulated collections of fat.
- Following sterile preparation and local anesthesia similar to above, a small (3–4 mm) punch is made through the skin and capsule into the lipoma (*Fig. 29.5*).
- The skin should be first stretched opposite the direction of the relaxed skin tension lines, so an oval forms after the punch is removed.
- Again, with firm digital pressure, the fat is squeezed out (*Fig. 29.6*).
- Closure is as above.

 Advantages:

- These procedures are simpler and less time consuming than full excision.
- Cosmetic results are similar to excision if lesion selection is appropriate.

 Caveats:

- As one is operating with a presumptive diagnosis, extruded material should be submitted for histologic examination.
- If a larger than anticipated dead space is encountered, the base of the wound can be included in the vertical mattress bites.
- Alternatively, the wound can be opened more widely to accommodate buried stitches to close off the dead space.

 References:

Hardin FF. A simple technique for removing lipomas. J Dermatol Surg Oncol 1982; 8:316–317.

Lieblich LM, Geronemas RG, Gibbs RC. Use of a biopsy punch for removal of epithelial cysts. J Dermatol Surg Oncol 1982; 8:1059–1062.

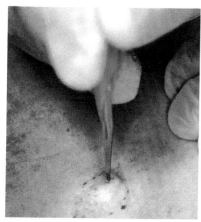

Fig. 29.1 Incision of cyst with a #11 blade. (From Salasche SJ, Winton GB, Adnot J. Surgical pearls. Dermatol Clin 1989; 7:75–110.)

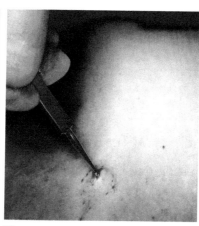

Fig. 29.2 Curette loosens cyst wall. (From Salasche SJ, Winton GB, Adnot J. Surgical pearls. Dermatol Clin 1989; 7:75–110.)

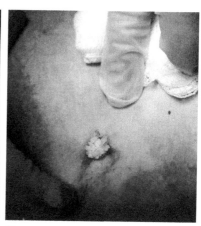

Fig. 29.3 Expression of cyst contents. (From Salasche SJ, Winton GB, Adnot J. Surgical pearls. Dermatol Clin 1989; 7:75–110.)

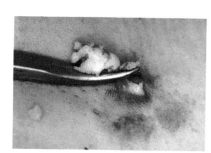

Fig. 29.4 Cyst wall extraction. (From Salasche SJ, Winton GB, Adnot J. Surgical pearls. Dermatol Clin 1989; 7:75–110.)

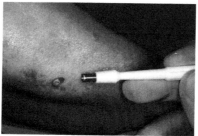

Fig. 29.5 Punch into lipoma. (From Salasche SJ, Winton GB, Adnot J. Surgical pearls. Dermatol Clin 1989; 7:75–110.)

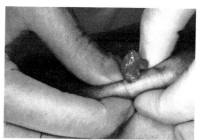

Fig. 29.6 Extrusion of fatty material. (From Salasche SJ, Winton GB, Adnot J. Surgical pearls. Dermatol Clin 1989; 7:75–110.)

Rationale:

- It is not uncommon for epidermoid or acne cysts to become inflamed and tender.
- They may resolve with combinations of warm compresses, antibiotics or intralesional injection of dilute corticosteroids (3–5% triamcinolone).
- In some instances, the cyst may drain intermittently, or become fluctuant, or the skin overlying may become very thin and attenuated (*Fig. 30.1*).
- In these instances, incision and drainage may be the best option.

Technique:

- A ring block of local anesthesia with 1–2% lidocaine with epinephrine is performed the area.
- The cyst or abscess should not be entered with the injection needle.
- A stab incision is then made into the cyst contents with a #11 or #15 surgical blade (*Fig. 30.2*).
- With lateral inward compression, the contents are expressed.
- Residual pockets are expressed by insertion and spreading of hemostat blades.
- Any residual cyst wall should also be removed with a hemostat or forceps.
- The cyst cavity is flushed with sterile saline under some pressure from a large-bore syringe (*Fig. 30.3*).
- Finally, the wound is loosely packed with an iodoform gauze wick to help drainage (*Fig. 30.4*).
- This is changed on a daily basis until cessation of drainage and second-intention healing is underway (*Figs 30.5 and 30.6*).
- Patients should be advised that a scar revision may be required several months after healing has settled down.

Advantage:

- This is more or less a last resort approach, but timely incision and drainage will offer the patient both relief from pain and the best chance for a good outcome.

Caveats:

- The wick requires daily changing.
- Most family members are unable to perform this task and office visits or arrangement for home visits are mandatory.

Reference:

Salasche SJ, Winton GB, Adnot J. Surgical pearls. Dermatol Clin 1989; 7:75–110.

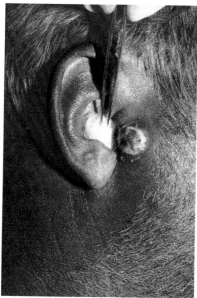

Fig. 30.1 Pre-auricular fluctuant tender cyst. Note cotton in ear canal. (From Salasche SJ, Winton GB, Adnot J. Surgical pearls. Dermatol Clin 1989; 7:75–110.)

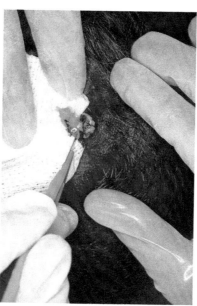

Fig. 30.2 Stab incision with a #11 scalpel blade. (From Salasche SJ, Winton GB, Adnot J. Surgical pearls. Dermatolol Clin 1989;7:75-110.)

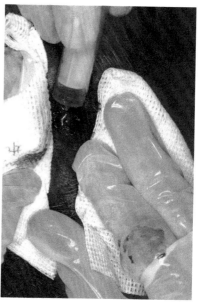

Fig. 30.3 Cavity flushed with sterile saline. (From Salasche SJ, Winton GB, Adnot J. Surgical pearls. Dermatol Clin 1989;7:75-110.)

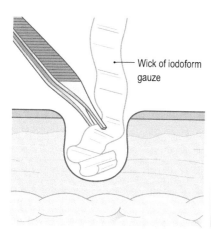

Wick of iodoform gauze

Fig. 30.4 Cavity loosely packed with iodoform gauze.

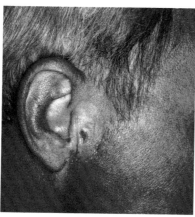

Fig. 30.5 Healing after 2 weeks.

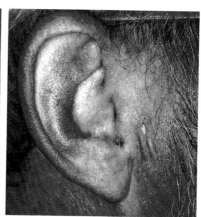

Fig. 30.6 Healing after 6 weeks.

Rationale:

- Shave or scoop excision is a frequently used modality for pigmented lesions.
- This is especially so for the removal of low-risk dysplastic lesions in a patient with many of them (*Fig. 31.1*).
- Periodically, the surgeon miscalculates the depth of the lesion and inadvertently transects it rather than removing it completely (*Figs 31.2 and 31.3*).
- If the lesion turns out to be a benign dysplastic nevus, blue nevus, Spitz nevus or other benign lesion, no harm has been done.
- On the other hand, if it turns out to be a melanoma and only the superficial shaved-off portion is submitted for examination, the prognostic information from having an accurate Breslow thickness is lost.
- Microstaging, assignment to risk group and possible need for sentinel lymph node biopsy are all dependent on Breslow thickness.
- In the event that such a problem arises, the authors recommend the following course of action.

Technique:

- As soon as it becomes apparent that the lesion has been transected, inform the patient and explain that the surgical plan has to be altered.
- Increase the scope of local anesthesia, bring out the surgical tray and perform a full-thickness elliptical excision of the residual lesion.
- Call the pathology laboratory and inform them of the situation.
- Speak with the technician/pathologist who will be blocking in the tissue and the pathologist who will be reading the tissue.
- This attention to detail will maximize the probability that the two pieces of tissue will be married up, examined appropriately and yield the appropriate parameters to further manage the patient.

Advantages:

- Obviously, patient welfare should be the prime directive in this type of situation.
- Failure to follow through to attain the needed diagnosis and parameters may adversely affect care.

Caveats:

- Full-thickness excision of the base of the lesion is better than attempting to remove it with another scoop shave.
- It will be easier for the pathologist to manage the two blocks of tissue.

Reference:

Salasche SJ, Grabski WJ. Clinical conundrum: transverse section of a pigmented lesion. Dermatol Surg 1997; 23:578–582.

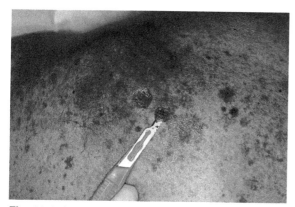

Fig. 31.1 Appropriately executed scoop excision; note peripheral rim of normal tissue and no pigment left in the biopsy site. (From Salasche SJ, Grabski WJ. Clinical conundrum: transverse section of a pigmented lesion. Dermatol Surg 1997; 23:578–582.)

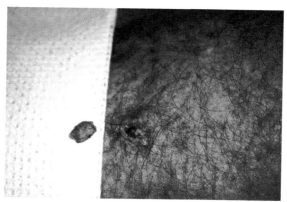

Fig. 31.2 Lesion transected. (From Salasche SJ, Grabski WJ. Clinical conundrum: transverse section of a pigmented lesion. Dermatol Surg 1997; 23:578–582.)

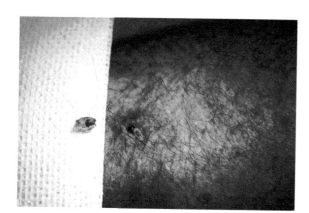

Fig. 31.3 Lesion transected; note pigment on undersurface of biopsy. (From Salasche SJ, Grabski WJ. Clinical conundrum: transverse section of a pigmented lesion. Dermatol Surg 1997; 23:578–582.)

Rationale:

- Visualization, counter-traction and stabilization are prerequisites to the performance of meticulous cutting, undermining and electrocautery.
- A surgical assistant can aid in securing all of these (*Fig. 32.1*).
- Special situations, such as a large epidermal cyst, a mobile ear keloid or the fragile skin of the proximal nail fold (See Tip 67) may be facilitated by the use of retraction sutures.
- Besides the advantages noted above, utilization of retraction stitches precludes the use of potentially damaging skin hooks or tissue forceps and fingers in the surgical field (*Fig. 32.2*).

Technique:

- After ring block anesthesia of the tissue around the cyst, an ellipse of redundant skin is drawn (*Fig. 32.3*).
- A 3-0 or 4-0 non-absorbable suture is placed into the center of the proposed excision.
- Care must be taken to secure a good dermal bite, but the cyst wall should not be entered or the keratinaceous material will leak out (*Fig. 32.4*).
- The suture is left long so the surgeon can manipulate the pull and direction of the cyst like a puppeteer (*Fig. 32.4*).
- By pulling in various directions the surgeon can apply counter-traction and expose any portion of the field he or she desires to dissect out and finally enucleate the intact cyst (*Figs 32.5 and 32.6*).

Advantages:

- The surgeon can control the amount of tension and direction on the retraction suture.
- Hence, exposure and counter-traction are facilitated without having to instruct an assistant.

Caveats:

- The suture must be placed precisely.
- If it is too superficial, it may rip out when upward tension is applied.
- It may enter the cyst itself if placed too deeply, causing the smelly, keratinaceous material to leak out.

Reference:

Salasche SJ, Orengo I. Surgical pearl: the retraction suture. J Am Acad Dermatol 1994; 30:118–120.

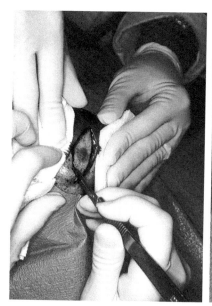

Fig. 32.1 Surgical assistant providing exposure and counter-traction.

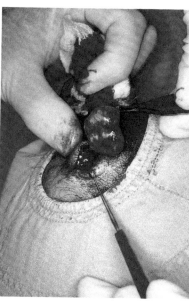

Fig. 32.2 Pilar cyst with fingers and instruments in field.

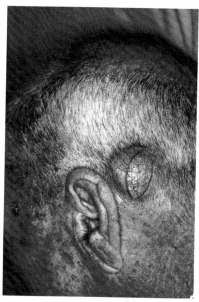

Fig. 32.3 Pilar cyst with proposed excision of extra skin. (From Salasche SJ, Orengo I. Surgical pearl: the retraction suture. J Am Acad Dermatol 1994; 30:118–120.)

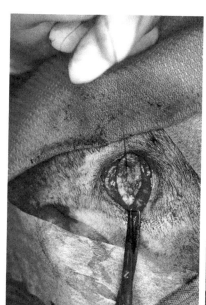

Fig. 32.4 Placement of retraction suture and initial dissection.

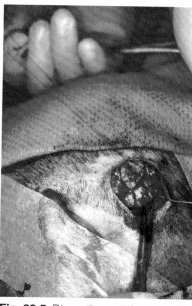

Fig. 32.5 Dissecting out the cyst with aid of retraction suture. (From Salasche SJ, Orengo I. Surgical pearl: the retraction suture. J Am Acad Dermatol 1994; 30:118–120.)

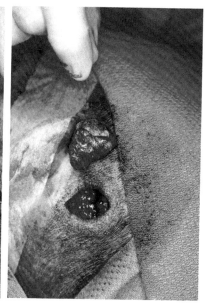

Fig. 32.6 Intact cyst completely enucleated.

Section 4
Flaps

Rationale:

- To understand flap design and tissue movement dynamics, a thorough knowledge of the components of the flap are required.
- A flap is a full-thickness segment of skin that is incised, elevated and moved (rearranged) about an attached pedicle to fill a nearby defect.
- Importantly, its viability is sustained by maintaining a portion of the original blood supply.
- Blood reaches the body of the flap through the vascular lifeline, the pedicle (or base), which remains attached to the contiguous skin (*Figs 33.1 and 33.2*).
- Axial flaps are supplied by a named artery. For example, the midline forehead flap is supplied by the supratrochlear artery.
- In random flaps, the blood supply reaches the body through the subdermal plexus of vessels.
- It is important not to undermine too far under the pedicle of a random flap.
- This increases mobility, but also the distance blood must flow to reach the most distal portion of the body.
- The blood flows upward through the subcutaneous fat in island pedicle flaps.

Technique:

- The defect to be repaired is known as the primary defect, while the one created by incising and elevating the body of the flap is the secondary defect (*Figs 33.1, 33.2, 33.3 and 33.4*).
- Primary movement is the movement of the body of the flap to fill all or a portion of the primary defect (*Fig. 33.5*).
- Secondary movement is the inward motion of all the surrounding tissue (after undermining) that helps close the primary and secondary defects (*Fig. 33.6*).
- Elasticity and mobility of the surrounding tissues determine the combination of primary and secondary movement required to close the defects.

Advantages:

- Knowing the 'language' of flaps helps understand how they are designed, how they survive and how to discuss aspects of 'flapology' with colleagues.

Reference:

Salasche SJ, Winton GB. Cutaneous surgical flaps: basic terminology and concepts. J Assoc Mil Dermatol 1988; 14:19–23.

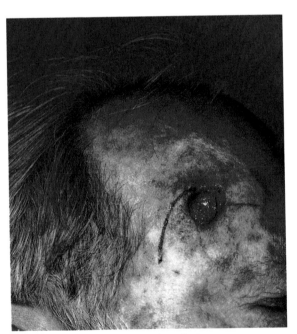

Fig. 33.1 Proposed rotation flap design.

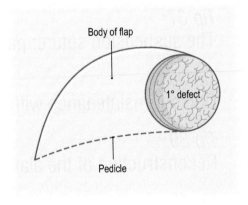

Fig. 33.2 Body, pedicle and primary defect.

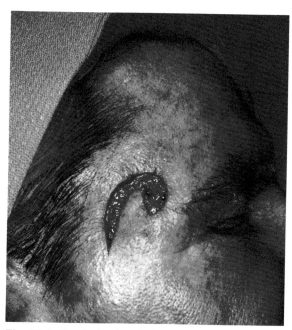

Fig. 33.3 Flap incised and elevated. Secondary defect created.

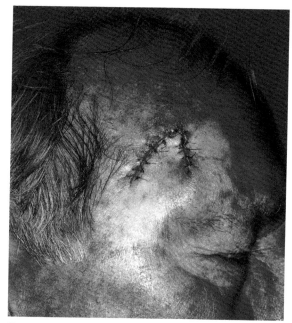

Fig. 33.4 Defect closed by combination of primary and secondary movement.

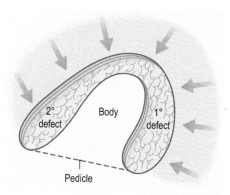

Fig. 33.5 Areas of proposed undermining around 2nd defect. Shaded area indicates the extent of undermining. Note that the pedicle is not undermined. Arrows indicate secondary movement to help close the 1st and 2nd defects.

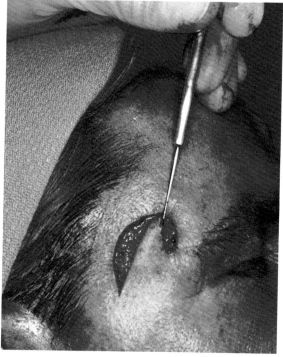

Fig. 33.6 Primary movement into primary defect.

Rationale:

- The tension vector (TV) of any type of closure is a very important concept to understand when performing repairs on the face.
- The TV may be defined as the summation of all the forces of tension of a closure expressed at a single point.
- Each type of closure has a TV, whether it be a primary elliptical closure, a flap or even the wound contraction attendant to second-intention healing.
- It is usually expressed with arrows (*Figs 34.3 and 34.5*).
- The greatest impact will be on free margins such as the eyelid, lip, eyebrow and nostril rim.
- Free margins are easily distorted as they offer little resistance to a pulling force (*Figs 34.2 and 34.3*).
- The consequence of a proposed closure TV can be tested beforehand with the use of a test stitch, toothed forceps or skin hooks (*Figs 34.2 and 34.4*).

Technique:

- Side-to-side closure TV is the easiest to identify as it is usually perpendicular to the line of closure, although, as will be seen, this can be modified by the surgeon to fit specific needs.

- Undermining and pretesting with skin hooks or placing a test stitch verifies the choice.
- In the first example, the vertical closure of the lower cutaneous lip defect pulls down the corner of the mouth (*Figs 34.1, 34.2 and 34.3*).
- On the other hand, redirecting the tension vector to a more advantageous transverse direction eliminates the problem (*Figs 34.4, 34.5 and 34.6*).

Advantages:

- Understanding the concept of the tension vector is a powerful tool in the decision-making process on how to repair a defect.
- It, along with other factors, such as where there is recruitable skin, the direction of the relaxed skin lines, how much of a cosmetic unit is affected and the effect of the proposed closure on symmetry, all help determine the best option.

Reference:

Salasche SJ, Jarchow RR, Feldman BD, et al. The suspension suture. J Dermatol Surg Oncol 1987; 13:973–978.

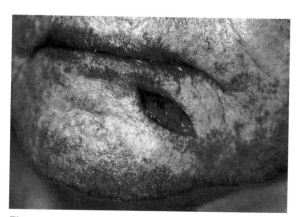

Fig. 34.1 Elliptical defect of cutaneous lower lip.

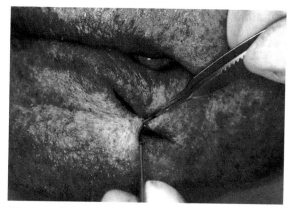

Fig. 34.2 Proposed closure pulls down corner of mouth.

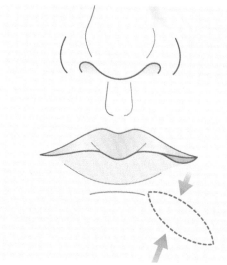

Fig. 34.3 Arrows indicate vertically oriented tension vector.

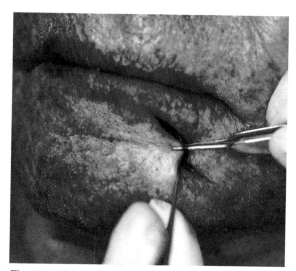

Fig. 34.4 Second proposed closure more advantageous.

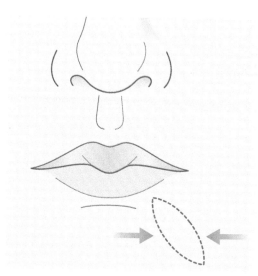

Fig. 34.5 Tension vector oriented in horizontal plane.

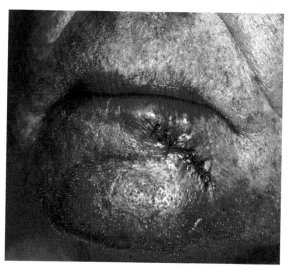

Fig. 34.6 Final closure using horizontal tension vector.

Tension Vector of Closure: Rotation and Advancement Flaps

 Rationale:

- The tension vector (TV) of a flap (tissue rearrangement) is more difficult to identify than that of a side-to-side closure.
- It is even more critical to understand them, as the stakes are higher with flaps.
- The tension vector varies for each type of flap pulled.
- Following are discussions of the two flaps that are pulled into place.

 Technique:

Rotation flap:

- The TV is fairly straightforward (*Figs 35.1, 35.2 and 35.3*).
- But notice in this closure the body of the flap is 'pulled' into the primary defect.
- Accordingly, one of the key differences from transposition flaps is that in rotation and advancement flaps, the primary defect is closed (partially or entirely) first.
- The point of maximal tension is at a point on the flap furthest from the pedicle (*Fig. 35.2*).
- Hence, the blood supply is at risk at this point.
- Because the flap is 'pulled' into place, it wants to recede back to where it came from.
- This contributes to the tension on the distal portion.
- Rotation flaps are at risk for distal necrosis.

Advancement flap:

- Another type of 'pulling' flap where the tissue is dragged into place.
- The maximal tension is also at a point furthest from the base or pedicle blood supply (*Figs 35.4, 35.5 and 35.6*).

 Advantages:

- Being able to identify the TV allows the surgeon to plan closures in an informed manner and hopefully avoid repairs that would result in cosmetic or functional disfigurement.
- An in-depth understanding of the TVs allows the surgeon to anticipate untoward effects of the proposed closure and adjust accordingly.

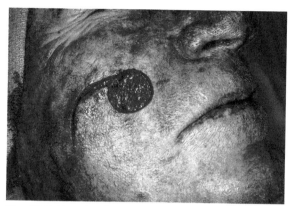

Fig. 35.1 Rotation flap design.

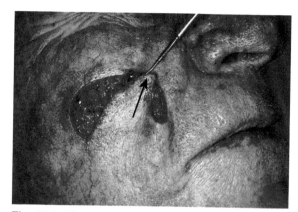

Fig. 35.2 Distal body of flap pulled into place. Arrow
indicates TV.

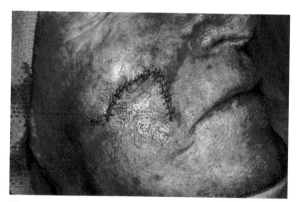

Fig. 35.3 Dog-ears removed and closure completed.

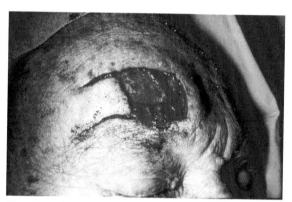

Fig. 35.4 Advancement flap design.

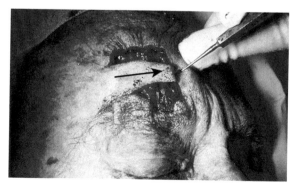

Fig. 35.5 Distal body of flap pulled into place. Arrow
indicates TV.

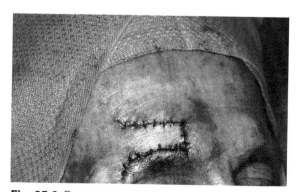

Fig. 35.6 Dog-ears removed and closure completed.

Determining the Final Scar Lines and Tension Vector of the Rhombic Flap

Rationale:

- It is often difficult to visualize beforehand what the final scar lines of the extremely useful but complicated rhombic flap design will look like.
- Predetermining this will allow the surgeon to place the scars in favorable skin tension lines or junction lines between cosmetic units and ensure that the venous and lymphatic drainage is positioned advantageously.
- Similarly, knowing the tension vector of closure will prevent creating functional or cosmetic deformities of free margins.

Technique:

- The classic rhombic flap is constructed by fashioning a four-sided diamond-shaped defect.
- It is a slightly tipsy equal-sided parallelogram with a long and short diagonal.
- The short diagonal is extended its exact length and a final line is drawn parallel and equal in length to the line of the rhomboid facing it (*Figs 36.1 and 36.2*).
- If one obliterates this last line and the parallel one opposite it, the proposed final scar line may be clearly visualized (*Fig. 36.3*).
- Once all the incisions are made and the flap elevated, the rhombic transposition flap is completed by initially closing the secondary defect (*Fig. 36.4*).
- The key stitch is from the last incision point made with the scalpel to where the short diameter was initially elongated beyond the rhombic defect (*Fig. 36.4*).
- All the forces of closure are concentrated at this point and therefore it defines the tension vector.

Advantages:

- This simple technique takes the guesswork out what is often a daunting conceptual problem for the inexperienced surgeon and makes a useful flap more accessible.
- The surgeon can predetermine the appearance of each of the possible configurations (*Fig. 36.5*).

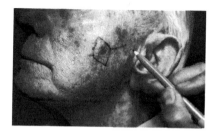

Fig. 36.1 Rhombic design with extension of the short diagonal.

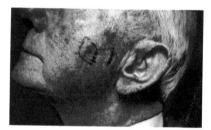

Fig. 36.2 Flap design completed.

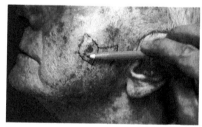

Fig. 36.3 Final scar lines visualized by eliminating final line and one opposite and parallel to it.

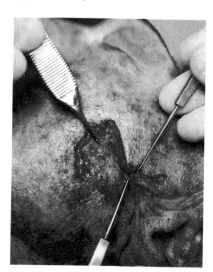

Fig. 36.4 Final configuration: skin hooks define tension vector.

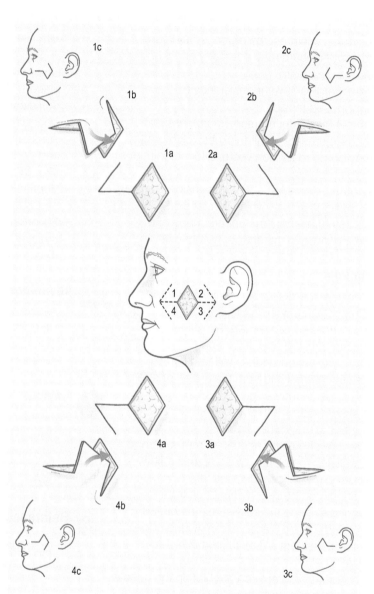

Fig. 36.5 All the possible configurations of this rhombic defect.

The Suspension Suture: Partial Closure of Defect Near Free Margin

 Rationale:

- In some instances, the proposed tension vector of closure may adversely affect one of the free margins.
- Free margins have no resistance to unopposed tension.
- Off-set bias suturing (see Tip 26), tissue rearrangements or full-thickness skin grafts may be good tension vector-altering solutions to the problem.
- Another alternative is the suspension ('tacking' or 'pexing') suture, which is a tension-reducing stitch that anchors the undersurface of a wound edge to the underlying periosteum.

 Technique:

- Consider the defect shown in *Figure 37.1*.
- Direct closure would pull up the free margin of the eyebrow to an elevated position asymmetric with the other side.
- The suspension stitch is initiated by taking a healthy dermal bite from the undersurface of the upper wound edge (*Fig. 37.2*).
- It should not extend superficially and cause a surface dimple when tied.
- The bite should be about 2–3 mm wide and parallel to the blood flow to preserve flow distally; in this location, vertically.
- It should be taken 5–7 mm back from the wound edge to insure that routine buried sutured can be placed at the wound edge after placement of the suspension suture (*Fig. 37.2*).
- The stitch is completed by rotating the needle down to bone and then upward to include a good bite of periosteum (*Fig. 37.2*).

- When secured, the wound is partially closed with all the tension directed to the periosteum and none to the free margin (*Fig. 37.3*).
- One or more suspension sutures may be placed.
- Sufficient buried sutures are then placed at the wound edges in a routine manner to insure eradication of dead space, wound eversion and gentle coaptation of the skin edges (*Fig. 37.4*).
- Routine closure is then completed with non-absorbable stitches (*Fig. 37.5*).
- Favorable bony sites include the frontal bone, the zygomatic arch, the malar eminence and the pre-maxilla (*Fig. 37.6*).

 Advantages:

- Allows side-to-side closure rather than more complicated flaps or grafts.
- Tissue is spared by not performing the more sophisticated procedures.

Caveats:

- Avoid injuring vital blood vessels and nerves with blind insertion of the anchoring bite.
- It is safer to spread the tissue with a fine-tipped hemostat until the periosteum is exposed.

 Reference:

Salasche SJ, Jarchow R, Feldman BD, et al. The suspension suture. J Dermatol Surg 1987; 13:973–978.

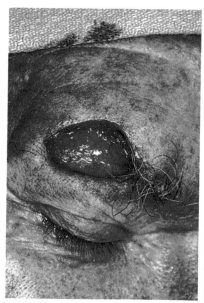

Fig. 37.1 Defect of right eyebrow and lower forehead.

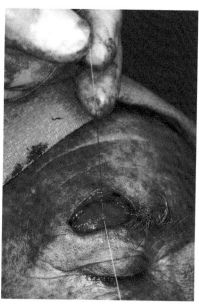

Fig. 37.2 Suspension suture in place. (From Salasche SJ, Jarchow R, Feldman BD, et al. The suspension suture. J Dermatol Surg 1987; 13:973–978.)

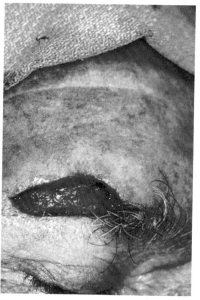

Fig. 37.3 Wound size halved. (From Salasche SJ, Jarchow R, Feldman BD, et al. The suspension suture. J Dermatol Surg 1987; 13:973–978.)

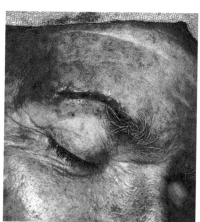

Fig. 37.4 Wound almost closed following placement of subcuticular stitches. (From Salasche SJ, Jarchow R, Feldman BD, et al. The suspension suture. J Dermatol Surg 1987; 13:973–978.)

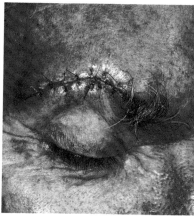

Fig. 37.5 Wound completed with interrupted surface stitches. (From Salasche SJ, Jarchow R, Feldman BD, et al. The suspension suture. J Dermatol Surg 1987; 13:973–978.)

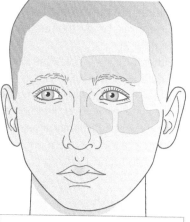

Areas best for pexing sutures

- Frontal bone
- Lateral orbital wall
- Side of nose/nasal bones
- Malar eminence/zygomatic arch

Fig. 37.6 Areas best suited for suspension sutures. (From Salasche SJ, Jarchow R, Feldman BD, et al. The suspension suture. J Dermatol Surg 1987; 13:973–978.)

Rationale:

- The repair of certain defects adjacent to cosmetic boundary lines may result in the loss of a natural concavity.
- This often involves defects of the nose (*Fig. 38.1*).
- A popular form of repair is to move extra cheek skin across the concavity of the nasofacial sulcus between the cheek and nose to the fill the nasal defect.
- As a result, tenting of the sulcus may occur, leading to loss of the contour and an asymmetric appearance (*Fig. 38.2*).
- The solution described below maintains the contour by using suspension sutures to recreate the concavity.

Technique:

- First, the tissue rearrangement design, either a cheek advancement or a crescentic advancement flap, is elevated and undermined (*Fig. 38.1*).
- Then an appropriate number of suspension sutures are placed into the periosteum of the pre-maxilla below the nasofacial sulcus (*Fig. 38.3*).
- Either 4-0 or 5-0 colorless non-absorbable suture or polyglactin (Vicryl) may be used.
- These are accomplished by taking a dermal bite parallel with the direction of flap movement sufficiently proximal to the wound edge to allow for anchoring into the periosteum and leaving sufficient room for the wound edge to advance easily and fill the defect.
- This should be apparent at the time the suspension sutures are snugged down and tied off (*Fig. 38.4*).
- The distal edge of the advancement is trimmed to just fit into the defect (*Figs 38.5 and 38.6*).
- Buried subcuticular stitches at the wound edge are placed and, finally, the surface sutures (*Figs 38.7 and 38.8*).

Advantages:

- With this technique, readily available redundant skin of the cheek can be moved across junction lines without causing a cosmetic distortion.
- An extra benefit is that much of the tension is directed down to the periosteum and not the distal edge of the flap.

Caveats:

- Correct placement of the suspension sutures to recreate the concavity is critical. If they do not reiterate the symmetric location of the sulcus, the benefit is lost.
- Insure there is sufficient tissue beyond the suspension suture to fill the defect.

Reference:

Salasche SJ, Jarchow R, Feldman BD, et al. The suspension suture. J Dermatol Surg 1987; 13:973–978.

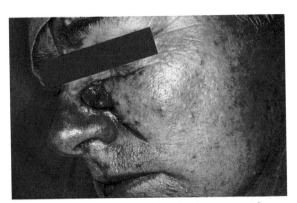

Fig. 38.1 Nasal defect with cheek advancement flap design.

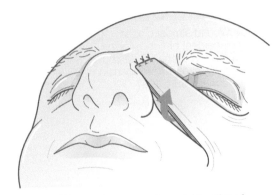

Fig. 38.2 Direct advancement would 'tent' and obliterate the concavity of the nasofacial sulcus.

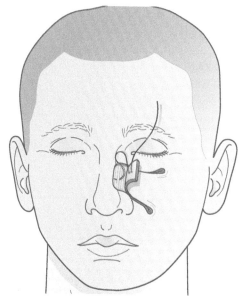

Fig. 38.3 Placement of the suspension suture.

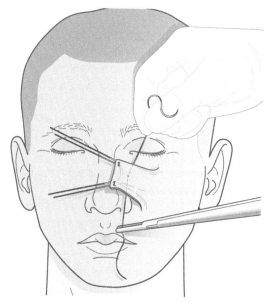

Fig. 38.4 Suspension sutures tied off.

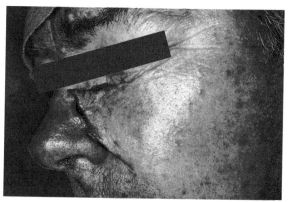

Fig. 38.5 Advancement flap pushed into place as suspension sutures are tied off. Note excess distal flap skin.

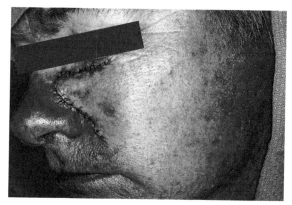

Fig. 38.6 Excess distal skin has been trimmed and the subcuticular and surface sutures are in place.

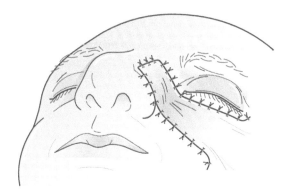

Fig. 38.7 Concavity maintained.

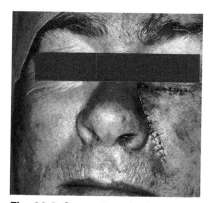

Fig. 38.8 Concavity maintained.

Rationale:

- The alar–facial–lip sulcus is the concavity created by the juncture of the alar base, medial cheek and uppermost cutaneous lip.
- This sulcus is very difficult to recreate when the tissue has been lost.
- During reconstruction of defects, it is easy to distort the region with poorly placed incisions.

Technique:

Reconstruction of the sulcus:

- Examine the intact contralateral side and use it as a mirror image model in planning the reconstruction.
- Evaluate the defect and see to what extent tissue is missing from each of the three areas: alar base, medial cheek and upper lip (*Fig. 39.1*).
- When feasible, design reconstructions individually for each of the three areas with their repairs meeting in the location of the initial sulcus.
- Sometimes, only one or two of these three units needs to be reconstructed, as the remainder can be left to heal by second intention because of its concave nature.

Reconstruction technique utilizing the tissue from this sulcus for repair of adjacent tissue loss:

- Incisions made medial to the upper end of the nasolabial line, for example with a perialar crescentic rotation/advancement flap, should not be made immediately at the reflection of the alar base but rather should be separated from the base by 1 or 1.5 mm (*Figs 39.1 and 39.3*).
- This leaves a small plateau into which newly advanced, rotated, or transposed tissue can then be secured without the potential problem of blunting of the alar base–upper lip groove.
- The perialar crescentic rotation/advancement flap borrows tissue from the upper lip/medial cheek/lower nasal sidewall to repair defects of the lower nasal dorsum or cutaneous upper lip (*Figs 39.3 and 39.4*).

Advantages:

- Efforts to maintain the normal anatomy of these three cosmetic units are rewarded with fine esthetic outcomes.
- Incisions placed just lateral to the reflection of the alar base are complicated far less frequently by the problems of maceration and/or delayed healing, as can be seen when incision is made directly in the reflection.

References:

Early JJ. Perialar extention and lip advancement in the closure of lip defects. Br J Plast Surg 1984; 37:50–54.

Webster JP. Crescentic perialar cheek excision for upper lip flap advancement with a short history of upper lip repair. Plast Reconstr Surg 1955; 16:434–464.

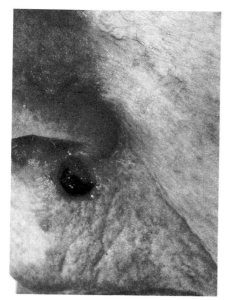

Fig. 39.1 Defect on cutaneous upper lip adjacent to sulcus.

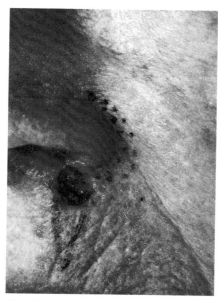

Fig. 39.2 Optimal location for an incision made through the alar–facial–lip sulcus is depicted with the dotted line just lateral to the alar base.

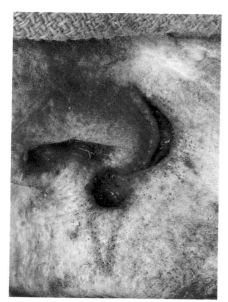

Fig. 39.3 Perialar crescentic rotation/advancement flap designed showing planned incisions (dotted lines) and areas to be excised (shaded areas).

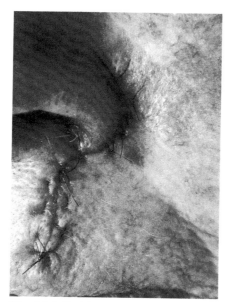

Fig. 39.4 Perialar crescentic rotation/advancement flap completed.

Rationale:

- Most wounds are optimally closed with adjacent tissue by either primary closure or adjacent tissue transfer (flap).
- Not infrequently, a situation arises where a circular defect will almost close, but the optimal direction of closure and what to do with the dog-ears are problematic.
- Here, three Burrow's triangles around the circle are removed, creating a final scar that resembles a carmaker emblem, hence the name Mercedes flap.
- It allows tissue advancement from three opposing directions around the wound.

 Technique:

- The wound is undermined at the level appropriate for the anatomic location.
- Three triangular Burrow's wedge-like excisions are outlined at approximately equal distances around the defect (*Fig. 40.1* Black tracings).
- The apex of the Burrow's triangles are oriented away from the central wound while the base of triangles sits on the edge of the defect and each should occupy approximately one-third of its circumference (*Fig. 40.1* white arrows, points, and dotted lines).
- The wound is diminished by placing sutures that connect the junctures of the base of each triangle.
- This can be accomplished by three separate buried absorbable stitches or a running circumferential buried stitch (*Figs 40.2 and 40.3*).
- The outlined triangles are then excised (*Fig. 40.4*).
- The wound is closed (*Figs 40.5 and 40.6*).

 Advantages:

- These flaps are very useful where the skin is thick such as on the scalp and trunk.
- The Mercedes flap is also very effective in thinner skin such as on the temple or the extremities.

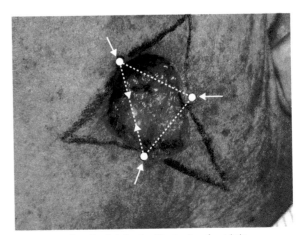

Fig. 40.1 Surgical defect with design for triple Burrow's triangle.

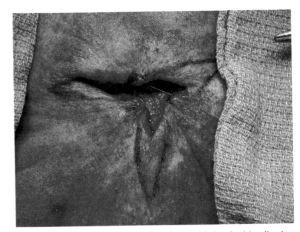

Fig. 40.2 Partial closure of defect with buried 'pulley' stitch.

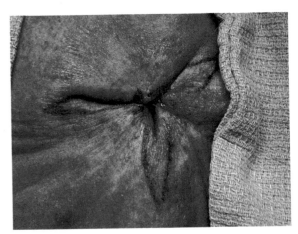

Fig. 40.3 Further closure of defect.

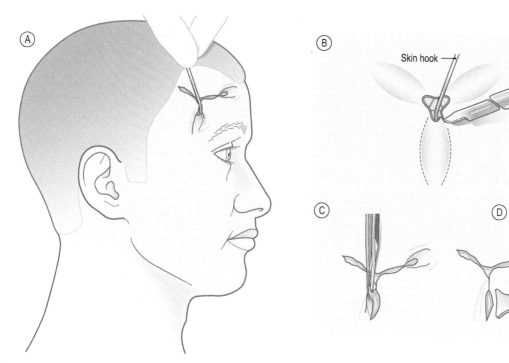

Fig. 40.4 Excision of Burrow's triangles.

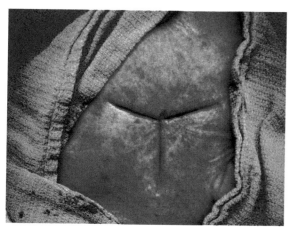

Fig. 40.5 Closure with buried stitches.

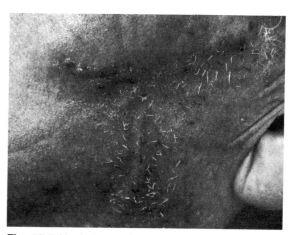

Fig. 40.6 Healed wound.

Section 5

Grafts

Rationale:
- Full-thickness skin grafts (FTSGs) are a frequently used reconstruction modality.
- Trimming the fat off the undersurface of the graft optimizes its revascularization.
- The graft should remain hydrated during this phase of the operation.
- Because it is kept wet, it is slippery (*Fig. 41.1*).
- Seceral tips help in this process.

Technique:
- Drape a sterile saline-soaked 4 × 4 gauze sponge over the dorsum of the index finger of the surgeon's non-dominant hand (*Fig. 41.2*).
- Place the graft fat-side up on the distal radial portion of this finger (*Fig. 41.2*).
- Secure the graft sides with pressure from the thumb and middle finger (*Fig. 41.3*).
- Using a blunt-tipped tissue scissors with the blades slightly opened, press down firmly until a small packet of fat protrudes upward between the blades (*Fig. 41.3*).
- The fat is snipped off and wiped away on an open portion of the gauze.
- The graft is rotated around so a fresh portion is presented over the convex surface.
- Care should be taken to include trimming of the very edge of the graft (*Fig. 41.4*).
- Trimming is continued until all the fat is removed and the white surface of the dermis is noted.

- The author's favorite scissors is the 4½ inch, fine dissecting, blunt-tipped Kaye tissue scissors (*Fig. 41.5*).
- One blade is serrated, which helps grasp and cut tissue.
- However, any sharp tissue scissors will work.

Advantages:
- This provides a secure, non-slip work area while keeping the graft moist.
- The convexity of the finger helps protrude the fat upward, facilitating the process.
- A convenient place to deposit the excess fat is provided.

Caveats:
- Aggressive trimming might lead to a buttonhole defect with consequent cosmetic sequences.
- The graft should remain hydrated with sterile saline throughout the procedure.

Reference:
Salasche SJ, Feldman BD. Skin grafting: Perioperative technique and management. J Dermatol Surg Oncol 1987; 32:863–869.

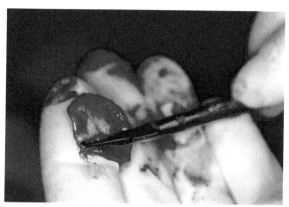

Fig. 41.1 Graft directly on gloved finger is unstable and slides around.

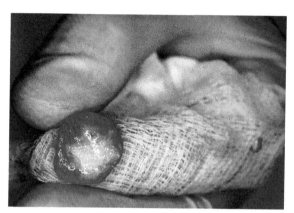

Fig. 41.2 Graft draped over wet gauze and secured by other fingers.

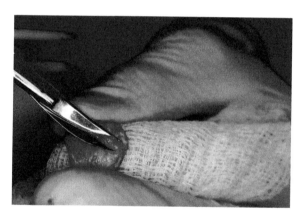

Fig. 41.3 Fat herniates up through scissor blades. (From Salasche SJ, Feldman BD. Skin grafting: Perioperative technique and management. J Dermatol Oncol 1987; 32:863–869.)

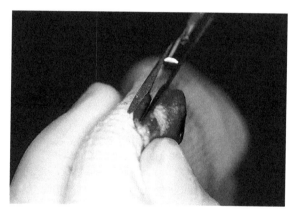

Fig. 41.4 Edges of graft are also trimmed.

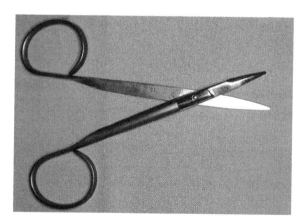

Fig. 41.5 Kaye scissors.

Freehand Harvesting of a Small Split-Thickness Skin Graft

 Rationale:

- Split-thickness grafts are usually chosen to cover a large defect, often in areas with poor vascularity.
- Sometimes, a small partial-thickness graft is required because a thin graft is required to match the site.
- Such a site is the nail unit, for example, following excision of a squamous cell carcinoma or Bowen's disease (*Fig. 42.1*).

 Technique:

- The donor site should be glabrous skin such as the ventral forearm, upper inner arm, abdomen, or, for the adventuresome, the lateral-most hypothenar area (the little finger-side edge of the palm).
- The donor site is marked to match the recipient site (*Fig. 42.2*).
- It is wise to oversize about 10% or so.
- Continue marking for an elliptical closure, taking the relaxed skin tension lines of the region into account.
- With the tip of a Bard-Parker #15 blade, score the graft donor site just into the reticular dermis around the entire perimeter (*Fig. 42.2*).
- The blade is then inserted into the dermis parallel and flat to the skin (*Fig. 42.3*).

- Once a pocket is developed, the entire graft can be incised by sliding the flat blade back and forth along the entire undersurface.
- While there is obviously no plane at this depth in the skin, staying at the same depth is relatively easy.
- Once this is done, the graft can be released by freeing the rest of the perimeter.
- After the graft is harvested, it can be sewn directly into the recipient site (*Fig. 42.4*).
- Returning to the donor site, the entire ellipse can be incised down to the desired subcutaneous level to include the apical tips and the remaining donor site dermis (*Fig. 42.5*).
- The defect is then repaired with a layered closure (*Fig. 42.6*).

 Advantage:

- Ability to secure a small, thin graft in a cosmetic manner.

 References:

Langtry JA. Small split-thickness skin graft technique harvested by score and shave technique. Br J Dermatol 2004; 68s:91–102.

Snow S, Zweibel S. Freehand skin grafts using the shave technique. Arch Dermatol 1991; 127:633–635.

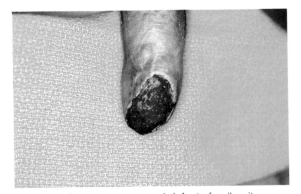

Fig. 42.1 Post-tumor removal defect of nail unit.

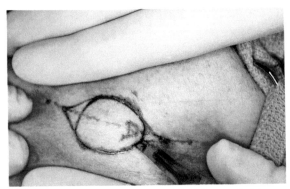

Fig. 42.2 Donor site, design and initial superficial scoring.

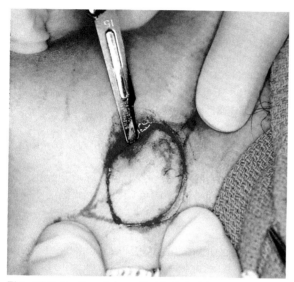

Fig. 42.3 Graft excision with blade held parallel with the skin surface.

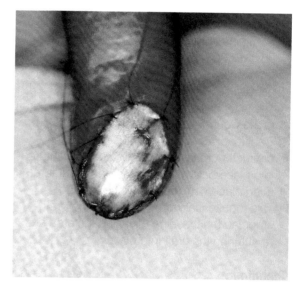

Fig. 42.4 Graft sewn into place.

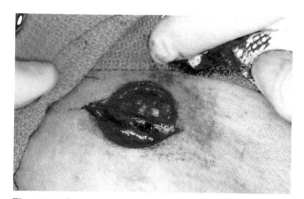

Fig. 42.5 Donor site converted to full-thickness ellipse.

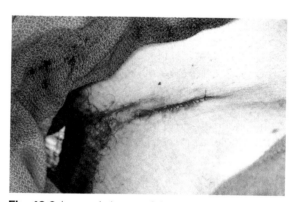

Fig. 42.6 Layered closure of donor site.

Basting Suture for Full-Thickness Skin Graft under Direct Visualization

 Rationale:

- Complete apposition of a full-thickness skin graft (FTSG) to the wound bed can be accomplished with either a tie-over bolster or basting sutures.
- The latter secure the central portion of the graft to the wound bed.
- Traditional technique dictates that the full perimeter of the graft be trimmed and sutured into place before placing the basting suture(s).
- Blind placement may result in bleeding.
- This requires taking down part of the graft, stopping the bleeding, cleaning the area and re-suturing the graft into place.

 Technique:

- This problem can be obviated by placing the basting sutures before all the perimeter sutures are completed.
- An arc of about one-third of the superior circumference is sutured into place (*Fig. 43.1*).
- The basting sutures can be placed under direct vision by inserting the needle through the surface of the graft and then taking a small but secure 'bite' into the graft recipient bed (*Fig. 43.2*).
- The suture is subsequently run back through the undersurface of the graft about 3–4 mm from the entry point (*Fig. 43.3*).

- It is then tied snugly into place (*Fig. 43.4*).
- After sufficient stitches are placed to insure complete apposition, the remainder of the perimeter of the graft is secured (*Fig. 43.5*).

 Advantages:

- Allows one to see the placement of each basting suture and easily correct any bleeding that may occur.
- If bleeding does occur, it can be managed without taking down the whole graft (*Fig. 43.6*).

 Caveats:

- Do not overtrim the graft; leave sufficient graft tissue to complete tension-free closure of the perimeter after securing the center with the basting suture(s).
- Otherwise, the graft will be pulled tight as a drum and away from the bed.

 Reference:

Adnot J, Salasche SJ. Visualized basting sutures in the application of full-thickness skin grafts. J Dermatol Surg Oncol 1987; 13:1326–1329.

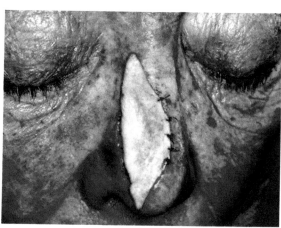

Fig. 43.1 One portion of the graft perimeter is secured. (From Adnot J, Salasche SJ. Visualized basting sutures in the application of full-thickness skin grafts. J Dermatol Surg Oncol 1987; 13:1326–1329.)

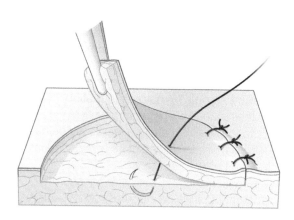

Fig. 43.2 Bite taken from wound bed after passed through graft. (Adapted from Adnot J, Salasche SJ. Visualized basting sutures in the application of full-thickness skin grafts. J Dermatol Surg Oncol 1987; 13:1326–1329.)

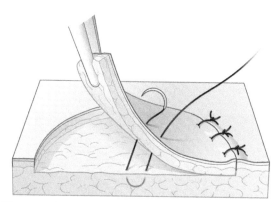

Fig. 43.3 Suture is run back up through undersurface of graft. (Adapted from Adnot J, Salasche SJ. Visualized basting sutures in the application of full-thickness skin grafts. J Dermatol Surg Oncol 1987; 13:1326–1329.)

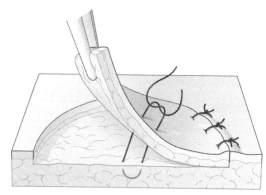

Fig. 43.4 Basting suture tied into place. (Adapted from Adnot J, Salasche SJ. Visualized basting sutures in the application of full-thickness skin grafts. J Dermatol Surg Oncol 1987; 13:1326–1329.)

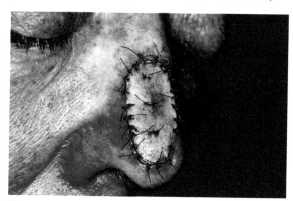

Fig. 43.5 After sufficient basting sutures are placed, the perimeter is secured. (From Adnot J, Salasche SJ. Visualized basting sutures in the application of full-thickness skin grafts. J Dermatol Surg Oncol 1987; 13:1326–1329.)

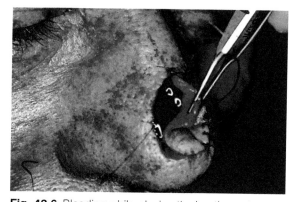

Fig. 43.6 Bleeding while placing the basting suture.

Continuous Tie-Over Bolster Dressings for Skin Grafts

Rationale:

- Tie-over bolster dressings are used to immobilize skin grafts and secure them uniformly over the recipient bed.
- They also help eliminate dead space and prevent seroma/hematoma formation.
- All these functions help graft survival.
- Historically, skin graft tie-over dressings have utilized multiple single suture ties placed into the graft edge.
- The multiple sutures are left long, and after placement of the bolster dressing the sutures are tied back and forth over the bolster (*Fig. 44.1*).
- This is a time-consuming and expensive (multiple sutures) technique.
- A continuous single suture run back and forth over the bolster and tied on itself offers a good alternative to the multiple suture technique.
- A variation on needle orientation described below may minimize blood flow compromise to the graft by the suture material.

Technique:

- The tie-over dressing is secured with a single running non-absorbable suture, usually 5-0 nylon, after the graft has been sutured in place.
- There are several potential patterns for securing the continuous tie-over dressing.
- The exact pattern of passes will depend on surgeon preference but all are predicated on using the soft, bulky bolster material (gauze or sponge) to help hold and direct the suture material.
- The suturing begins as a single standard skin suture with the needle passing perpendicular to the graft margin and with the short end left approximately 2.5 cm long (*Fig. 44.2*).
- In continuous fashion, the long portion of suture is then passed back and forth over the dressing with sufficient number of passes to adequately secure the bolster (2–4 passes usually suffices) (*Figs 44.3 and 44.4*).
- The final pass is brought back to the initial suture, after looping it under an earlier pass, and tied over the top of the dressing (*Fig. 44.5*).

- Each entry of the needle is just several millimeters peripheral to the skin graft edge and does not actually enter the skin graft.
- Whenever possible, the needle is directed in a perpendicular instead of parallel fashion to the graft edge, thereby minimizing any compromise to blood coming into the site from peripheral to the graft (*Fig. 44.6*).

Advantages:

- This is a rapid, secure and cost-effective technique to secure tie-over dressings.
- The perpendicular needle placement modification should allow maximal blood flow to reach the healing graft.

References:

Adams DC, Ramsey ML, Marks DJ. The running bolster suture for full-thickness skin grafts. Dermatol Surg 2004; 30:92–94.

Skouge JW. Letter to the editor. The running bolster suture for full-thickness skin grafts. Dermatol Surg 2004; 30:1180–1181.

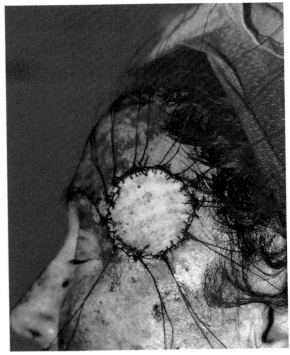

Fig. 44.1 Classic tie-over dressing with multiple single sutures.

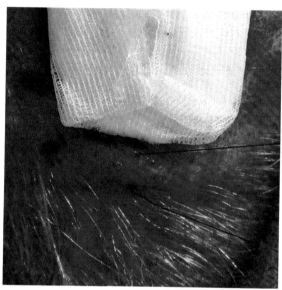

Fig. 44.2 First bite of tie-over suture with direction perpendicular to the wound.

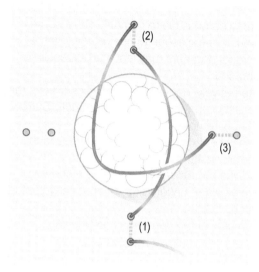

Fig. 44.3 Initial passes of tie-over dressing with continuous running non-absorbable suture.

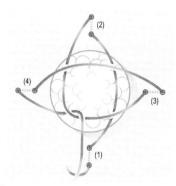

Fig. 44.4 One possible pattern for continuous tie-over dressing.

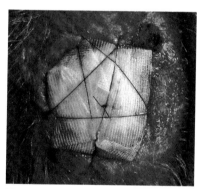

Fig. 44.5 Completed tie-over dressing.

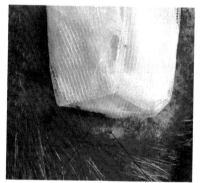

Fig. 44.6 First pass of tie-over suture with suboptimal (parallel) needle orientation to graft edge.

Rationale:

- It may be possible to primarily close some circular defects, but routine removal of the residual dog-ears may leave an excessively long scar.
- Alternatively, dog-ears on convex surfaces may persist even with seemingly adequate Burrow's triangle removal.
- This is because the collagen bundles in the dermis, instead of lying flat, tend to form a rigid rod-like protuberance, similar to a sheath of wheat, when bundled up within an enveloping stitch.
- Removal of the dog-ear as an M-plasty resolves both these problems.

Technique:

- The circular defect is undermined and the long axis of closure is determined (*Fig. 45.1*).
- One or two buried subcuticular stitches are placed at the middle of the wound to clearly define the compressive buckling that appears at each apex (the dog-ears).
- A skin hook or toothed forceps is used to elevate and exactly define the entire dog-ear (*Fig. 45.2*).
- As a reference point, the midpoint of the tissue upheaval closest to the skin edge is marked (ARROW, see *Fig. 45.2*, tip of scalpel) with a surgical marker.
- It will be used later as the apex of the three-corner stitch.
- With the skin hook in place, the periphery of the dog-ear is marked with curvilinear lines on each side from the wound edge to halfway around the dog-ear (*Fig. 45.2*).
- Note that in routine hockey stick Burrow's

triangle dog-ear repair, one or the other side would be chosen and the design carried all the way around the dog-ear mound. Here, we go half around both sides.
- Each side is then scored with a scalpel and incised full thickness with a tissue scissors, creating an apron of skin (*Fig. 45.3*).
- Care is taken to cut 90 degrees to the mound as it erupts from the skin, so it actually looks as though one is cutting at 60 degrees.
- The portion under the released apron of skin is further undermined if needed (*Figs 45.3 and 45.4*).
- The two 'wings' that have been liberated are then draped over the wound edges and again marked, scored and cut (*Figs 45.5, 45.6 and 45.7*).
- A three-corner stitch then completes the dog-ear removal with formation of an M-plasty (*Fig. 45.8*).

Advantages:

- Shortens the final scar.
- This improves appearance and in some instances negates crossing anatomic boundary lines.
- Accounts for dog-ears that would continue over convex surfaces.

Caveat:

- Try to put arms in or parallel to the relaxed skin tension lines.

Reference:

Salasche SJ, Roberts LC. Dog-ear correction by M-plasty. J Dermatol Surg Oncol 1984; 10:478–482.

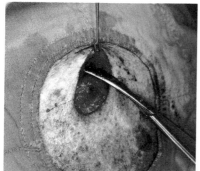

Fig. 45.1 Circular defect undermined.

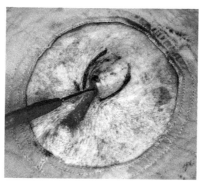

Fig. 45.2 Central stitches placed and dog-ear mound defined and outlined halfway on each side. (From Salasche SJ, Roberts LC. Dog-ear correction by M-plasty. J Dermatol Surg Oncol 1984; 10:478–482.)

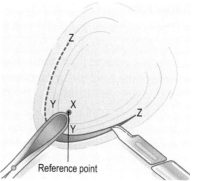

Fig. 45.3 Incise full thickness on each side.

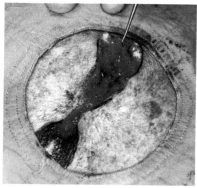

Fig. 45.4 Apron of skin elevated. (From Salasche SJ, Roberts LC. Dog-ear correction by M-plasty. J Dermatol Surg Oncol 1984; 10:478–482.)

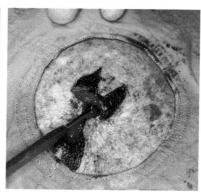

Fig. 45.5 Apron draped over wound and excess tissue marked for excision. (From Salasche SJ, Roberts LC. Dog-ear correction by M-plasty. J Dermatol Surg Oncol 1984; 10:478–482.)

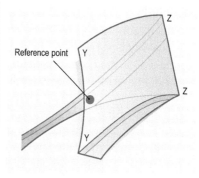

Fig. 45.6 Same as Figure 45.5.

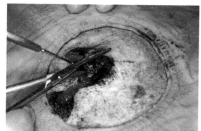

Fig. 45.7 Wings of excess tissue excised from both sides. (From Salasche SJ, Roberts LC. Dog-ear correction by M-plasty. J Dermatol Surg Oncol 1984; 10:478–482.)

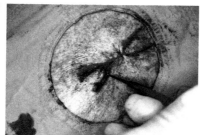

Fig. 45.8 Three-cornered stitch settles in the M-plasty.

Rationale:

- The surgical removal of a skin tumor often results in a defect that involves portions of two or more adjacent cosmetic subunits.
- One of the principles of modern reconstruction is to repair each subunit individually if possible.
- This preserves the naturally occurring junction or boundary lines between the subunits.
- As a corollary, these repairs often involve incisions into these boundary lines to help mobilize sufficient tissue to fill a portion of the defect.
- This paradigm works well because the naturally occurring boundary lines hide surgical scars well as they are the anticipated lines and shadows of the face.

Technique:

- Consider the defect in *Figures 46.1 and 46.2* which involves portions of the ala nasi, lateral side wall of the nose, cheek and upper lip.
- The surgical plan involves a relaxing incision under the alar base to repair the cutaneous upper lip and a crescentic cheek advancement flap to repair the cheek defect (*Fig. 46.3*).
- To accomplish the latter procedure, incisions are made along the nasofacial junction and the melolabial fold (*Fig. 46.3*).
- As the tissue is brought across toward the nose, Burrow's triangles or crescents of excess dog-ear tissue develop superiorly and inferiorly (*Fig. 46.3*).
- Once the triangles are removed and the lip is closed, the cheek flap is developed and inset into the nasofacial and melolabial contour lines (*Fig. 46.4*).
- Instead of discarding the Burrow's triangles, the portion from the melolabial fold is defatted and placed into the sidewall/alar defect as a full-thickness skin graft (*Fig. 46.5*).
- If all works well, the defect is obliterated and all scar lines fall within the natural junction lines of the face (*Fig. 46.6*).

Advantages:

- This rather complicated procedure is really quite efficient in terms of not using distant tissue such as a midline forehead flap.
- Instead, it makes use of tissue that would be normally discarded.
- It follows modern precepts of repairing individual subunits and utilizes adjacent skin with similar color and texture.

Caveat:

- If the graft fails, be prepared to allow the area to heal by second intention before attempting another repair.

References:

Chester EC. The use of dog-ears as grafts. J Dermatol Surg Oncol 1981; 7:956–959.

Kim KH, Gross VL, Jaffe AT, Herbst AM. The use of the melolabial Burrow's graft in the reconstruction of combination nasal sidewall–cheek defects. Dermatol Surg 2004; 30:205–207.

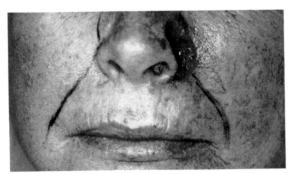

Fig. 46.1 Defect involving nose, lip and cheek: frontal view.

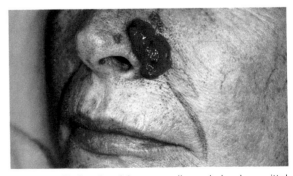

Fig. 46.2 Defect involving nose, lip and cheek: sagittal view.

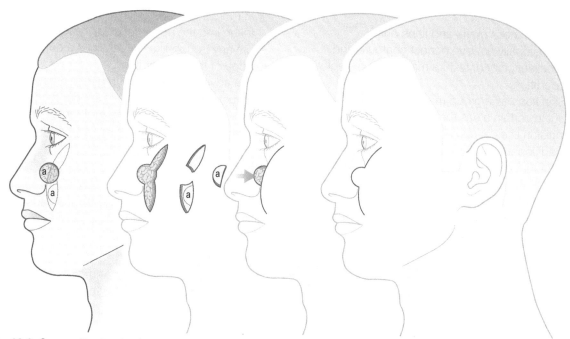

Fig. 46.3 Crescentic cheek advancement flap and development of Burrow's dog-ears.

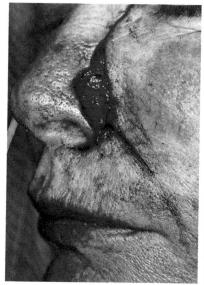

Fig. 46.4 Upper lip repaired and cheek advancement in place.

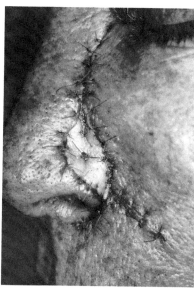

Fig. 46.5 Graft placed to fill nasal defects.

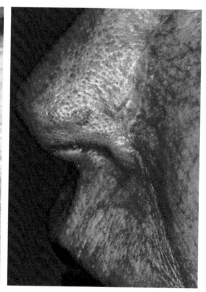

Fig. 46.6 Final healing.

Manual Dermabrasion of Full-Thickness Grafts and Flaps

Rationale:

- Full-thickness grafts and flaps only occasionally achieve perfect contours and excellent color or texture match with a single operation.
- Skin flaps as a group match better than grafts but in certain areas they may leave suboptimal incision lines or contour changes.
- Traditional dermabrasion to blend color and contour is done with a powered, hand-held tool that requires significant skill and special equipment.
- In addition, it aerosolizes blood, which may pose a risk to medical personnel.
- Having a simpler and safer alternative would be beneficial.

Technique:

- Manual dermabrasion can be done with sterile silicon carbide sandpaper (80–220 grade) or sanding screen in patches of about 5 × 5 cm (*Fig. 47.1*).
- The sanding can be done with either finger pressure or by wrapping the sandpaper around a 3 cc syringe and using that as a tool (*Fig. 47.2*).
- The graft or flap and surrounding 1 cm of tissue are prepped, outlined and infiltrated with 1% lidocaine with epinephrine (*Fig. 47.3*).
- Then, manually abrade the skin graft or flap and surrounding tissues until contours are evened (*Fig. 47.4*).
- Abrading the surrounding skin is necessary to blend the repair site with the adjacent skin.
- In most areas, the abrasion is taken down to the papillary dermis with fine bleeding points becoming visible (*Fig. 47.5*).

- In more sebaceous skin, this may need to be taken into the upper reticular dermis to smooth out any trough-like depressions around the edge of the graft or flap.
- It is advisable to start with gentle pressure and adjust pressure to achieve the depth required to even the contour of the graft or flap to the surrounding skin.

Advantage:

- This is a rapid, effective, safe and inexpensive way to dermabrade skin grafts and flaps to achieve optimal esthetic outcome.

Caveats:

- If done on only part of the nose, in particular part of a sebaceous nose, the dermabraded area will be smoother when compared to the other nonsanded areas.
- When the sanding will create side-to-side differences on the nose, it is appropriate to discuss with the patient the possibility of doing a more extensive bilateral dermabrasion.
- When sanding the nasal tip and supratip, one needs to balance sanding too little with only partial improvement versus sanding too much and making the cartilage too visible.

Reference:

Zisser M, Kaplan B, Moy RL. Manual dermabrasion. J Am Acad Dermatol 1995; 33:105–106.

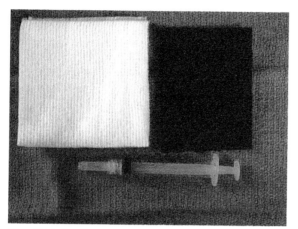

Fig. 47.1 Sterile silicone carbide sandpaper square.

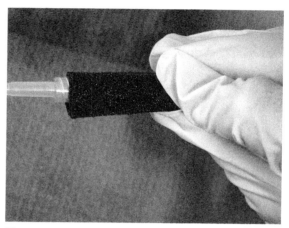

Fig. 47.2 Sterile silicone carbide sandpaper wound around 3 cc syringe.

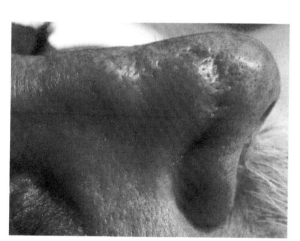

Fig. 47.3 Six weeks postoperative: bilobe flap with contour difference from flap fullness and incision line depression compared to surrounding skin.

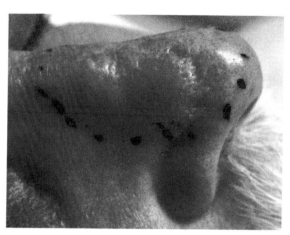

Fig. 47.4 Area to be sanded noted with dotted lines.

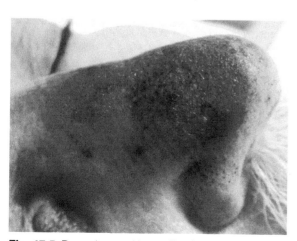

Fig. 47.5 Dermal wound immediately post-dermabrasion.

Rationale:

- Despite performing skilled surgical repairs, some scars do not mature as expected and are cosmetic liabilities.
- The scar itself may be rough, ragged, inflamed raised or depressed.
- There may be residual stitch marks around the scar.
- Most frequently, full-thickness skin grafts may have contour and/or color differences from the surrounding skin.
- Based on experience from performing superficial dermabrasion on post-traumatic scars to improve appearance, the same techniques have been applied to postsurgical scars.
- The procedure is best performed about 6 weeks postsurgery, as the molecular remodeling wound healing mechanisms are already in place.
- The sebaceous areas of the nose and forehead respond the best.

Technique:

- A good example would be the track marks left on either side of a scar when working on sebaceous skin or when the stitches are left in place too long (*Fig. 48.1*).
- The area is prepped and anesthetized.
- Using a hand engine (Osada) with a bullet- or pear-shaped diamond fraise, the area is lightly abraded to pinpoint bleeding.
- The entire area on each side of the scar is included (*Fig. 48.2*).
- Only pressure is used for hemostasis, not electrosurgery.
- Wound care is daily dressing changes and application of a petrolatum-based ointment and non-adherent dressing.

- Improved appearance may be expected within 2 weeks.
- For full-thickness skin grafts, light dermabrasion to the entire graft and feathered out for several millimeters of surrounding normal skin (for even blending) will often dramatically improve the appearance of the graft (*Figs 48.3–48.5*).

Advantages:

- Improved cosmetic appearance with a minimally invasive procedure.
- It is often wise to inform full-thickness graft patients at the time of initial surgery that they may require a touch-up dermabrasion in about 6 weeks.

Caveats:

- When dermabrading grafts, care should be taken not to abrade too deeply, particularly around the scar line of the graft.
- This may tend to accentuate the demarcation between graft and normal skin instead of improving appearance.

Variations:

- Lasers have been used for the same purpose.
- Manual dermabrasion with mesh screen is also effective (Tip 42).

References:

Nehal KS, Levine VJ, Ross B, et al. Comparison of high-energy pulsed carbon dioxide laser resurfacing and dermabrasion in the revision of surgical scars. Dermatol Surg 1998; 24:647–650.

Robinson JK. Improvement of the appearance of full-thickness skin grafts with dermabrasion. Arch Dermatol 1987; 23:1340–1345.

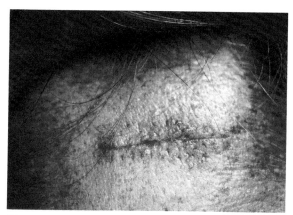

Fig. 48.1 Stitch marks on either side of scar following cyst removal.

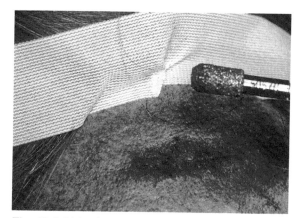

Fig. 48.2 Light dermabrasion to entire scar and surrounding skin.

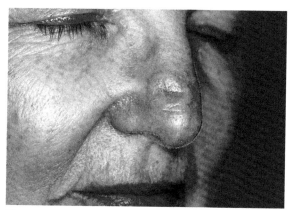

Fig. 48.3 Full-thickness skin graft with contour elevation.

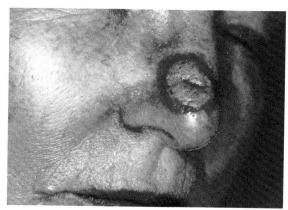

Fig. 48.4 Post abrasion.

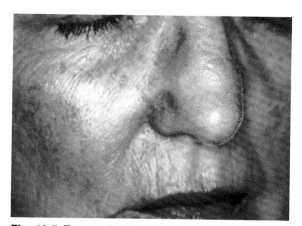

Fig. 48.5 Ten months later.

Section 6

Safety

Rationale:

- An orderly surgical tray and surgery room environment reflects on the surgeon in terms of safety, competence and overall attitude toward patient care.
- This includes simple things such as training personnel not to place surgical instruments on the surgical drapes even temporarily where they may fall off (*Fig. 49.1*).
- Or have bottles, especially open ones, between the operating field and the electrocautery unit where extending the connecting wire may cause a spill (*Fig. 49.2*).
- But it is the surgical tray that requires the most vigilance and effort to maintain in an orderly manner.
- The safety risks engendered by a poorly organized tray include injury and possible infection from needles, scalpel blades and skin hooks covered by used gauze pads (*Fig. 49.3*).

Technique:

- Depending on one's surgical practice, it may be convenient to have one generic surgical tray or several specialized trays for different types of surgery.
- For example, a hair transplant or liposuction tray will require different instruments and set-up than when performing Mohs' micrographic surgery (*Fig. 49.4*).
- Regardless, the key is to start with all instruments, syringes, gauze pads, cotton-tipped applicators (CTAs) and other equipment clearly visible and in a standardized place.
- The goal is to maintain this organized, open field so that everything on the tray remains clearly visible and easily/safely retrievable.
- Unnecessary materials, soiled gauze pads, suture packets, used CTAs should be appropriately discarded as the surgery progresses and not returned to the tray.

- Instruments should be removed and replaced to the appropriate place on the tray by the surgeon or assistant who is using them.
- In general, instruments should not be passed from hand to hand between personnel to decrease risk of sharps injury.
- In general, instruments should point away from the surgeon's hand, and all should point in the same direction.
- If someone is assisting, a neutral zone can be established and the assistant's instruments (suture scissors, skin hooks, etc.) can be arranged separately across a neutral zone.
- Several commercially available tray organizers are available to help maintain order (*Fig. 49.5*)
- One particularly important item to keep track of and maintain in a clearly visible state is the used suture needles.
- There are a variety of methods of doing this, but all rely on a standard, agreed plan.
- These include the spot provided on a commercial organizer, a gauze pad placed in a standardized corner of the tray or a designated place on a cloth covering the surgical tray holder (*Figs 49.6, 49.7 and 49.8*).

Advantages:

- Safety, safety, safety.
- Careful planning in this arena reflects on the surgeon's concern for the safety of the patient and the operating personnel, as well as his or her leadership ability.

Caveat:

- Keep it simple, consistent and ongoing.

Reference:

Trizna Z, Wagner RF. Surgical pearl: preventing self-inflicted injuries to the dermatologic surgeon. J Am Acad Dermatol 2001; 44:520–522.

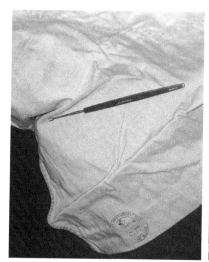

Fig. 49.1 Skin hook on edge of drape about to fall to the floor.

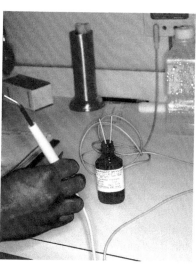

Fig. 49.2 Bottle of gentian violet about to stain the floor.

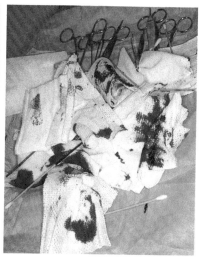

Fig. 49.3 Bloody gauze pads obscuring instruments on surgical tray.

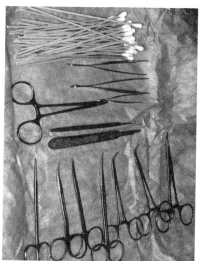

Fig. 49.4 Set-up for excisional surgery.

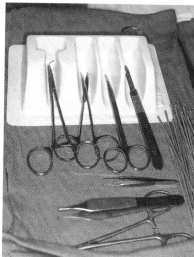

Fig. 49.5 Commercial surgical tray organizer.

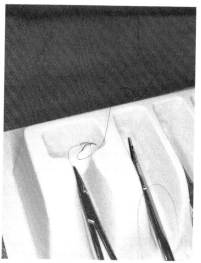

Fig. 49.6 Used needles in designated spot on plastic organizer.

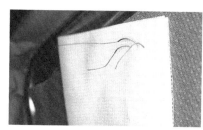

Fig. 49.7 Used needles arrayed together on gauze pad.

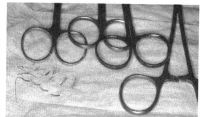

Fig. 49.8 Used needles placed in orderly manner in designated place of sterile covering of surgical tray.

Rationale:

- Unfortunately, a messy surgical tray increases the risk of needlestick injuries, which in turn increase the risk of transmission of HIV or hepatitis (*Fig. 50.1*).
- However, using a tool already on the tray, the medicine cup, the same end result can be achieved without an increase in expense.

Technique:

- When assembling surgical trays, include two glass or plastic medicine cups.
- One cup can be used to store saline or antiseptic solution to clean the surgical site.
- The other cup can be used to store the sharps.
- Once the tray is in use, lay one of the medicine cups on its side and place all the sharp instruments in the cup (*Fig. 50.2*).
- The blade handle with the blade, used blades, the needle holder with suture attached, used suture and the syringe with the local anesthesia are all stored in this cup.
- When surgery is finished, place used knife blades, cautery tips, syringe needles and suture needles in the cup and pour directly into the sharps container (*Fig. 50.3*).

Advantages:

- Using the medicine cup to store sharps is an easy habit to get into and does not require any special equipment or expense.
- The surgeon and assistants always know the location of sharps and at the end of the procedure the sharps can be disposed of easily in the larger sharps container.
- The biggest benefit of this pearl is that it is one way to decrease the unnecessary accidental needlestick injuries and subsequent trips to the occupational health department.

Reference:

Bell KA, Orengo I. Surgical pearl: behold the lowly cup. J Am Acad Dermatol 2002; 47:940–941.

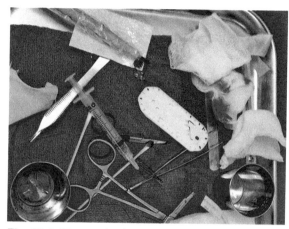

Fig. 50.1 Disorganized surgical tray.

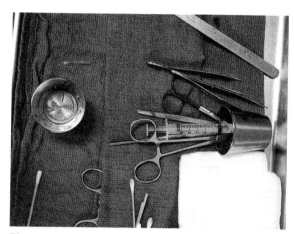

Fig. 50.2 Sharps while in use in cup.

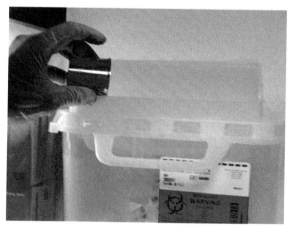

Fig. 50.3 Dumping sharps into container.

Rationale:

- At the end of a surgical procedure there is material that needs to be disposed of in a safe and efficient manner.
- Most of the emphasis and concern has been rightfully directed at disposal of the 'sharps'; suture and anesthetic needles and scalpel blades that could conceivably transmit communicable diseases (see Tips 49 and 50).
- However, bloody gauze sponges and suture packaging should also be disposed of properly (*Fig. 51.1*).

Technique:

- This maneuver can be carried out by either the surgeon or the assistant.
- A quick, novel approach is to gather up all this loose material in one gloved hand and, with the other gloved hand, pull it over the waste material (*Figs 51.2 and 51.3*).
- The maneuver is completed by then pulling the second glove over the waste packet (*Figs 51.4 and 51.5*).
- Finally, it is deposited safely in a hazardous waste container (*Fig. 51.6*).

Advantage:

- Nice, tidy, disciplined approach to a necessary chore.

Caveat:

- Make sure that all the 'sharps' are accounted for before picking up untidy and scattered soft material.

Reference:

Kimyai-Asadi A, Jih MJH, Goldberg LH, et al. Surgical pearl: a rapid sanitary technique for surgical waste control. J Am Acad Dermatol 2004; 50:642–643.

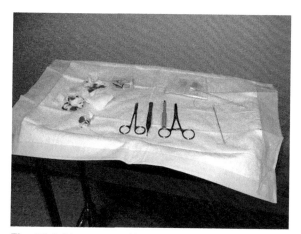

Fig. 51.1 Messy tray with bloody sponges.

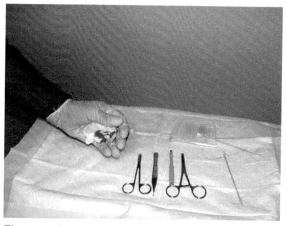

Fig. 51.2 Gathering contaminated material in one gloved hand.

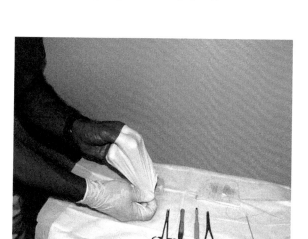

Fig. 51.3 Pulling glove over waste material like sleeve.

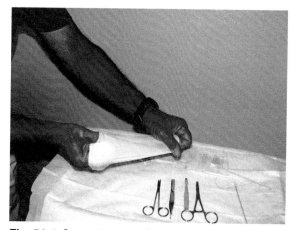

Fig. 51.4 Second glove pulled over to make secure packet.

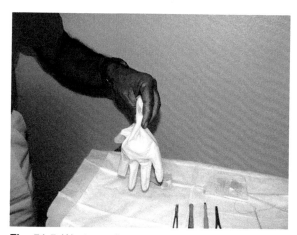

Fig. 51.5 Waste packet.

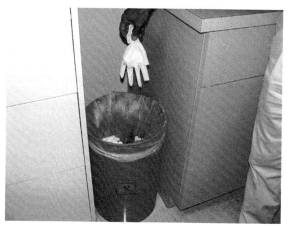

Fig. 51.6 Disposed in hazardous waste container.

Rationale:

- Periocular surgery, especially on the eyelid margins, requires measures to protect the cornea and globe.
- This applies equally for cold steel as well as laser surgery.
- There are many varieties and sizes of commercially available eye shields (*Fig. 52.1*).
- Surgical shields are usually plastic and are opaque or translucent.
- They are inserted with a suction cup applicator or by utilizing the molded handle.
- Laser shields are made of non-reflective stainless steel.

Technique:

- Initially, the eye is anesthetized with several drops of proparacaine hydrochloride 0.5% solution (*Fig. 52.2*).
- The inner concave surface of the shield, which will be in contact with the ocular globe, is then lubricated with ophthalmic antibiotic ointment.
- The shield is then grasped by the molded handle with a forceps or with the suction cup applicator (*Fig. 52.3*).
- The patient is asked to look upward while the lower eyelid is manually retracted.
- The shield is then slid in under the retracted lid (*Fig. 52.3*).
- The patient then reverses gaze and the shield is slipped into place under the opposite lid (*Fig. 52.4*).
- Removal after the procedure is a reversal of steps (*Fig. 52.5*).
- The importance of the shield in cancer surgery of the eyelids cannot be overemphasized (*Fig. 52.6*).

Advantages:

- The cornea and globe are protected.
- The surgeon is not distracted or worried about the cornea with the shield in place.

Caveats:

- The topical anesthesia may last 15–30 minutes after the shield is removed.
- Patients should be cautioned not to rub their eyes as there will be decreased sensation and risk of corneal abrasion.

Reference:

Wheeland RG, Bailin PL, Ratz JL, et al. Use of scleral eye shields for periorbital laser surgery. J Dermatol Surg Oncol 1987; 13:156–158.

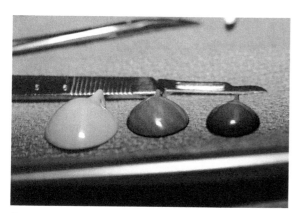

Fig. 52.1 Selection of corneal shields.

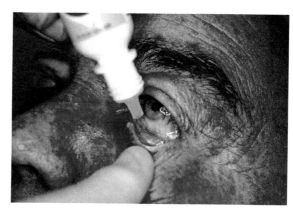

Fig. 52.2 Topical anesthesia of cornea.

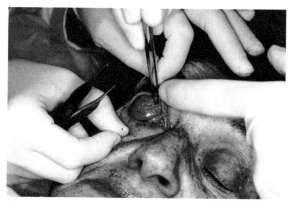

Fig. 52.3 Insertion of corneal shield.

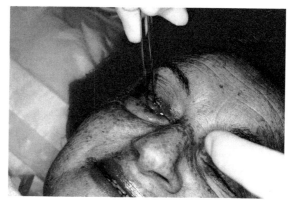

Fig. 52.4 Insertion completed.

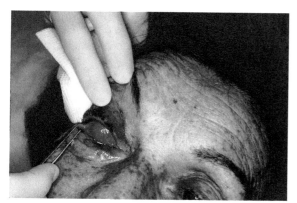

Fig. 52.5 Removal of shield.

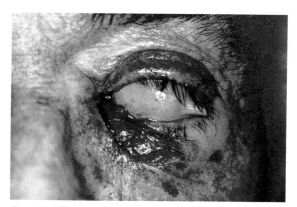

Fig. 52.6 Extensive tissue removal: shield protects globe.

TIP 53
Safety
The Sheathed Syringe

Rationale:

- Safety in the operating suite is of paramount importance to the operating team as well as the patient.
- An area of ongoing concern is the danger of needlesticks resulting from recapping of syringes (*Figs 53.1 and 53.2*).
- The danger of transmission of HIV and hepatitis B and C is a real threat to surgical personnel.
- During the performance of Mohs micrographic surgery, supplemental or repetitive local anesthesia may be necessary between stages and prior to the next stage.
- Uncapped needles should not be allowed on the surgical tray.
- Capping them is dangerous (*Fig. 53.2*).
- Several methods of 'safe' recapping have been devised but the benefits of commercially available resheathable syringes offer the safest alternative.

Technique:

- The SAFETY-LOK by Becton Dickinson (BD) is an example (*Fig. 53.3*).
- With the large-gauge needle that comes attached to the syringe, draw up the anesthetic fluid of choice (*Fig. 53.4*).
- Replace existing needle with a ½ or ¼ inch, 30-gauge needle.
- Inject the patient with local anesthetic prior to the initiation of surgery.
- Perform surgical excision.
- Between stages, the sheath is pulled down over the needle (*Fig. 53.5*).
- When pulled as far distally as it can go, the sheath completely covers and protects the needle point (*Fig. 53.6*).
- If more anesthesia is needed, slide the sheath back down to its original position and inject.

- At the completion of the procedure, pull the sheath all the way distally again, but this time twist or rotate the sheath on the barrel.
- This will permanently lock the sheath in the extended, safe position.
- The entire syringe can then be safely discarded into the appropriate safety receptacle.

Variants:

- There are various commercially available cap holding devices.
- These hold the cap up vertically and firmly so the syringe with needle can be inserted safely into the cap.
- Or a large forceps can be placed on its side.
- The cap with opening up is pushed into the 'V' of the forceps (*Fig. 53.7*).
- When anesthesia is complete, the needle is inserted into the cap and snapped into place (*Fig. 53.8*).

Advantages:

- Allows multiple-use injections of anesthesia safely from one syringe.
- More expensive, but cost is lessened if bought in bulk.

Caveat:

- Be sure not to twist or rotate the sheath in the extended position before the completion of surgery as it cannot be used once locked.

References:

Katz KH, Maloney ME. Surgical pearl: safely recapping needles during surgery. J Am Acad Dermatol 2002; 46:93–94.

Trizna Z, Wagner R. Surgical pearl: preventing self-inflicted injuries to the dermatologic surgeon. J Am Acad Dermatol 2001; 44:520–522.

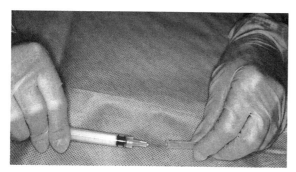

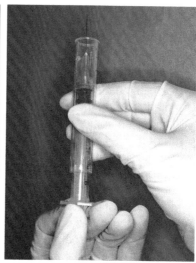

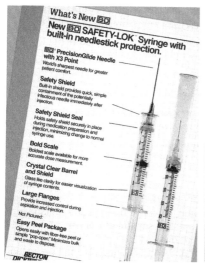

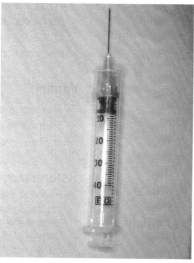

Fig. 53.1 Dangerous needle recapping.

Fig. 53.2 Demonstration of why needle recapping is hazardous.

Fig. 53.3 Sheathed syringe package. **Fig. 53.4** Sheathed syringe. **Fig. 53.5** Sheathing the needle.

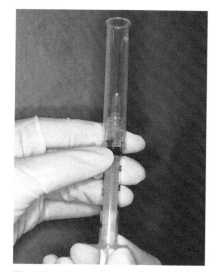

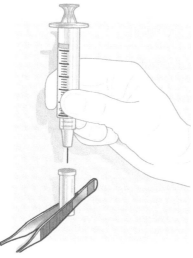

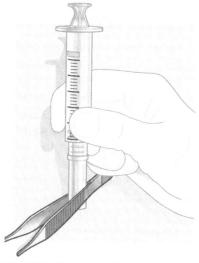

Fig. 53.6 Sheathing completed and safe between surgical stages.

Fig. 53.7 Needle cap placed in 'V' of forceps. (Redrawn from Katz KH, Maloney ME. Surgical pearl: safely recapping needles during surgery. J Am Acad Dermatol 2002; 46:93–94.)

Fig. 53.8 Needle safely snapped into place. (Redrawn from Katz KH, Maloney ME. Surgical pearl: safely recapping needles during surgery. J Am Acad Dermatol 2002; 46:93–94.)

TIP 54

Geometric Pattern Excision for Histologic Margin Control of Tumors

Rationale:

- Routine pathology processing of excised skin tumors by any of the standard techniques cuts the tissue perpendicular to the margin (bread-loaf).
- This examines less than 10% of the surgical margin including depth (*Fig. 54.1*).
- Some tumors, such as lentigo maligna or infiltrating basal cell carcinoma, have indistinct borders and variable subclinical extensions.
- Complete examination of the surgical margins would help to prevent local recurrences.

Technique:

- Instead of performing a standard elliptical or circular excision to remove the tumor, a geometric pattern, such as a triangle, square, rectangle or rhomboid, is designed that includes an appropriate margin around the tumor (*Fig. 54.2*).
- The excision should extend downward to an appropriate uniform depth within the subcutaneous tissue, so the plug of tissue removed is of equal thickness throughout.
- On a cutting surface and with a sharp #15 or #10 Bard-Parker scalpel, 2–3 mm wide vertical strips are cut parallel with each lateral margin (*Fig. 54.3*).
- These strips can be processed face up so the entire cut surface can be examined 'en face.'
- After each of the edges is cut, the remaining tissue can be turned over and the undersurface examined histologically for the adequacy of the deep margin.
- The tissue is embedded in paraffin blocks for routine processing and staining.
- Frozen section processing is feasible also.
- For proper orientation, the tissue should be color coded or marked with sutures, and a corresponding map should be drawn (*Fig. 54.4*).
- If a tumor is found on permanent sections, directed further excision is performed.

Advantages:

- A logical approach to margin control when the tumor borders are indistinct.
- A disadvantage is delayed closure.
- This technique has application when Mohs' micrographic surgery is not available.
- After confirming clear margins, geometric defects are amenable to closure with any number of tissue rearrangement designs.

Caveat:

- This technique requires participation of a dermatopathologist to coordinate correct embedding and blocking of tissue and interpretation of the processed slides.

Variant:

- The 'square' procedure, where only the peripheral strips are initially excised and the central area excised only at the time of closure.

References:

Johnson TM, Headington JT, Baker SR, et al. Usefulness of the staged excision for lentigo maligna and lentigo maligna melanoma: the 'square' procedure. J Am Acad Dermatol 1997: 37:758–764.

Prieto VG, Argenyi ZB, Barnhill RL, et al. Are en face frozen sections accurate for diagnosing margin status in melanocytic lesions. Am J Clin Pathol 2003; 120:203–208.

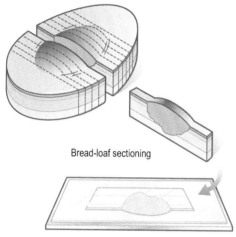

Fig. 54.1 Bread-loaf sectioning only samples some peripheral margins.

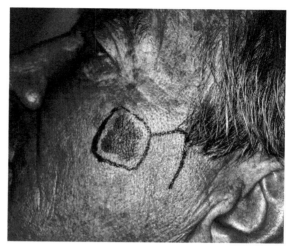

Fig. 54.2 Geometric excision design for lentigo maligna.

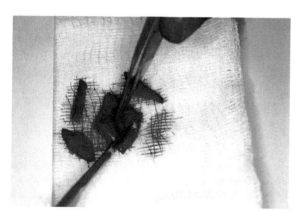

Fig. 54.3 Cutting en face peripheral strips.

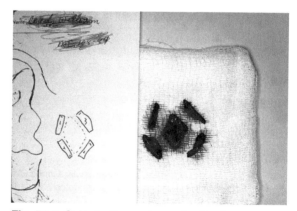

Fig. 54.4 Color coding and mapping the tissue.

Control of the Surgical Lamp: in the Best Light

Rationale:

- Surgeons frequently need to adjust the overhead lamp during surgery.
- Gloves become contaminated by touching the lamp handle or sides.
- The lamp itself can become contaminated by bloody gloves.
- This is not a problem when there is an extra assistant who is not part of the operating team.

Technique:

- There are commercially available disposable handle covers for specific lamp handles.
- To avoid the expense, a couple of innovations from material at hand solve the problem.
- The first is to attach a sterile or disposable glove to the lamp handle depending on the type of procedure being performed (*Fig. 55.1*).
- The other even simpler method utilizes the sterile gloves packet (*Fig. 55.2*).
- When the surgeon puts on his gloves, the surrounding sterile wrapping is left on the flat surface of the patient drapes or counter top.
- This can be used by the surgeon to rearrange the light as desired (*Fig. 55.3*).

Advantage:

- Simple solutions to a recurring situation.

Reference:

Ammirati CT. Aseptic technique. In: Robinson JK, Hanke CW, Sengelmann RD, et al., eds. Surgery of the skin: procedural dermatology. Philadelphia: Elsevier-Mosby; 2005:25–36.

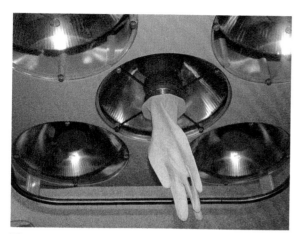

Fig. 55.1 Glove draped over the lamp handle.

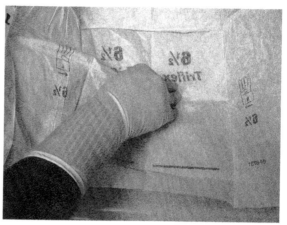

Fig. 55.2 Sterile glove wrapping. (Courtesy of Carl Vincuella, MD.)

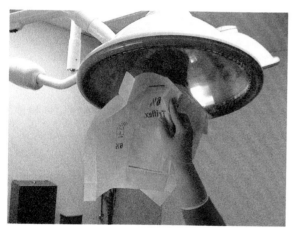

Fig. 55.3 Wrapping used to adjust surgical lamp. (Courtesy of Carl Vincuella, MD.)

Rationale:

- The Hyfrecator electrosurgical unit (ConMed Corporation) is a commonly used instrument in office procedures for hemostasis and in curettage and electrodesiccation (*Fig. 56.1*).
- Many of these procedures are 'clean,' but not sterile.
- Some surgeons prefer to place the pencil handpiece end of the unit on the surgical field.
- However, it can drop to the floor if left loose or spill the entire surgical tray if it has been fastened to it in some manner.
- Another problem is that when bloody gloved hands touch the unit, it becomes contaminated and must be cleaned between procedures.
- Both problems can be overcome by two simple aides.

Technique:

- To keep the handpiece and cord out the way, a plastic hook with an adhesive backing can be placed along the side of the mounted or mobile unit (*Fig. 56.2*).
- In either case, it should be within easy reach of the surgeon or assistant.

- The surgeon can remove it when needed and then secure it back to the hook when it is not needed.
- There are commercially available disposable non-sterile or sterile 'sleeves' (*Figs 56.1, 56.3 and 56.4*)
- Alternatively, a sleeve can be fashioned from a sterile or non-sterile ½ inch Penrose drain (*Fig. 56.5*).
- Or a very low-tech sheath can be made with a sterile or disposable glove (*Fig. 56.6*).
- The tip is fed through a finger of the glove and the needle-tip punched through when the end of the finger is encountered.

Advantages:

- The hook allows the handpiece and cord to be secured in a safe, but easily retrievable place.
- The protective sheath guards again external contamination of the electrocautery unit.

Reference:

Ammirati CT. Aseptic technique. In: Robinson JK, Hanke CW, Sengelmann RD, et al., eds. Surgery of the skin: procedural dermatology. Philadelphia: Elsevier-Mosby; 2005:25–36.

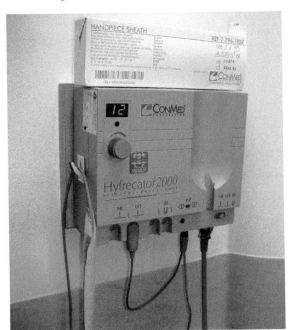

Fig. 56.1 Hyfrecator with disposable sheaths. (Courtesy of Carl Vincuella, MD.)

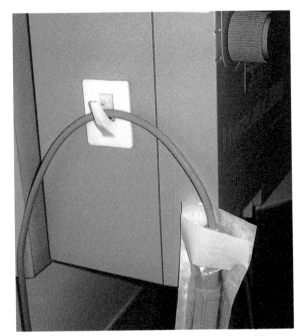

Fig. 56.2 Note the plastic hook on side of machine. Sheath in place. (Courtesy of Carl Vincuella, MD.)

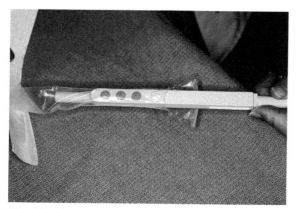

Fig. 56.3 Inserting pencil handpiece into sheath.

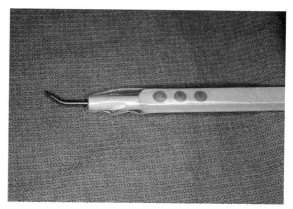

Fig. 56.4 Tip exposed.

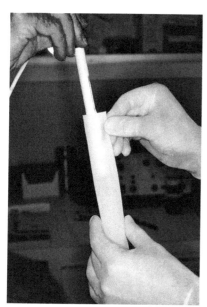

Fig. 56.5 Penrose drain as protective sheath.

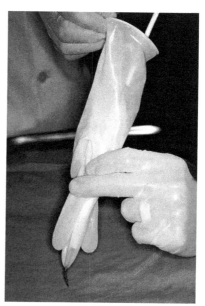

Fig. 56.6 Surgical glove used as protective sheath.

Section **7**

Instruments

Instruments for Special Occasions
The Mini-Scalpel System

Rationale:
- Surgical situations arise in certain locations that require small, delicate, sharp instruments.
- These include the nail unit, ear, lip and eyelid.

Technique:
- A useful acquisition is the 4-inch hexagonal or round knurled Beaver handle (*Fig. 57.1*).
- The small Beaver or MSP blades fit into a slot on the top, which screws down to tighten.
- The # 67 Beaver blade is a miniature version of the common #15 Bard-Parker blade (*Fig. 57.2*), while the # 64 Beaver blade has a useful rounded cutting tip (*Fig. 57.1*).
- Personna Gem and MSP have comparable mini-blades that work in the same handle.
- These blades are useful in constricted areas where precise, delicate cutting is required.
- This includes biopsies and excisions on the nail unit and lip (*Figs 57.3 and 57.4*).
- On the ear, paring of chondrodermatitis nodularis chronica helicis (CNCH) or removal of 'dumbbell'-shaped earlobe keloids is facilitated by the small cutting system (*Figs 57.5 and 57.6*).
- Obviously, there are numerous other innovative applications.

Caveat:
- The blades dull more quickly than standard blades.

Reference:
Leffell DJ, Brown MD, eds. Surgical instruments. In: Manual of skin surgery: a practical guide to dermatologic procedures. New York: Wiley-Liss; 1997:102.

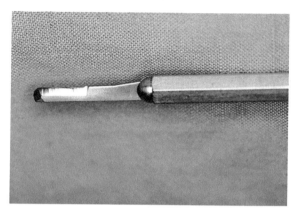

Fig. 57.1 Round-tip cutting surface of # 64 blade.

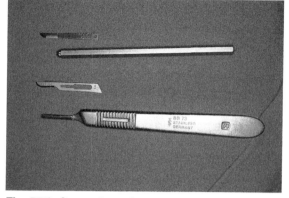

Fig. 57.2 Comparison of systems.

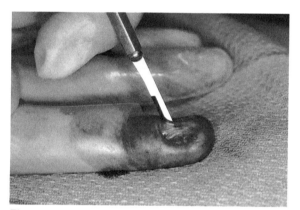

Fig. 57.3 Incision biopsy of nail unit.

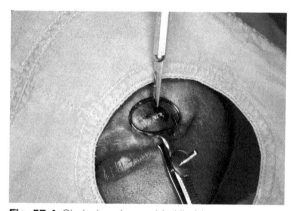

Fig. 57.4 Chalazion clamp-aided lip biopsy.

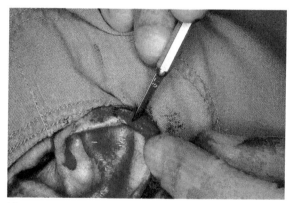

Fig. 57.5 Paring the damaged cartilage in CNCH.

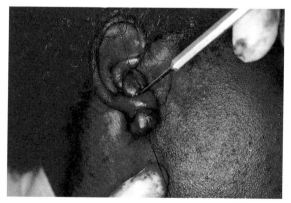

Fig. 57.6 Keloid of ear.

Rationale:

- Some lesions, because of their larger width, shallow nature or regional location, lend themselves to exquisitely precise excision utilizing the razor blade.
- Essentially, the technique involves either a shave biopsy or shave excision.
- The blade has found good application in removing benign intradermal nevi, seborrheic keratoses, epidermal nevi and flat warts.
- Macular or barely palpable pigmented lesions including junctional nevi and some dysplastic nevi are amenable to excision with a razor blade.
- Many razor blades are applicable; the authors have most experience with Wilkinson and Gillette blades.
- The Gillette Super Blue Blade is made of carbon steel and is extremely strong, sharp and flexible.
- It has a 1^{-6} inch cutting edge coated with a bacteriostatic agent, zinc naphthanate, and an anticorrosive agent.
- Autoclaving does not diminish the sharpness.
- According to personal preference, the surgeon may use the whole blade or cut it in half (as shown in the illustrations).

Technique:

- The blade can be adjusted for contour, width and depth.
- Bowing the blade only slightly allows a wide, shallow excision (*Fig. 58.1*).
- Increasing the bow results in a narrower and, depending on what is required, deeper excision (*Fig. 58.2*).
- The ends of the blade can be held with either the thumb and index finger or the thumb and middle finger using the index finger for better balance (*Figs 58.1 and 58.2*).
- The surrounding tissue can be stabilized and counter-traction applied by stretching or pinching with the non-surgical hand (*Fig. 58.3*).
- Epidermal lesions such as wide, thick seborrheic keratoses can be shaved flush by holding the blade relatively flat and cutting with a sawing motion (*Figs 58.3 and 58.4*).
- Any residual tissue can be curetted with a curette, or even the side of the razor blade using a flicking motion.
- For pigmented lesions, the blade can be bowed to meet the need for sufficient depth to get around the lesion (*Figs 58.5 and 58.6*).
- It is also a good idea to mark the perimeter of the proposed excision with a surgical marker to minimize potential local anesthesia related distortion.

Advantage:

- Very inexpensive 'boutique' cutting tool for special situations.

Caveats:

- Obviously, with so much exposed cutting edge, particular care should be taken during surgery and when disposing of the blades.
- If one cuts through a deeper than expected pigmented lesion and still has a portion of the lesion in the skin, remove the remaining portion with a full excision.

Reference:

Grabski WJ, Salasche SJ, Mulvaney MJ. Razor-blade surgery. J Dermatol Surg Oncol 1990; 16:1121–1126.

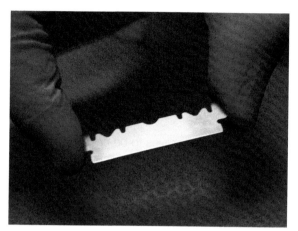

Fig. 58.1 Blade held flat and wide.

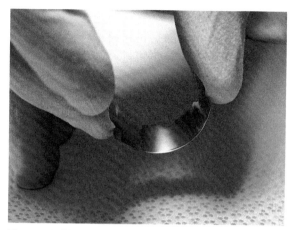

Fig. 58.2 Blade held bowed and narrow.

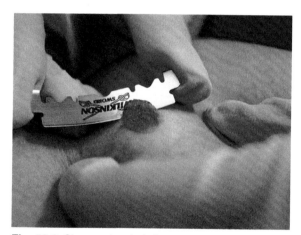

Fig. 58.3 Shave seborrheic keratoses.

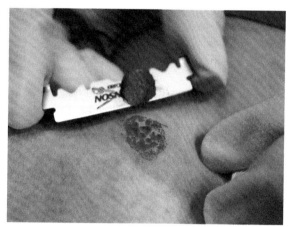

Fig. 58.4 Compete shave flush with skin.

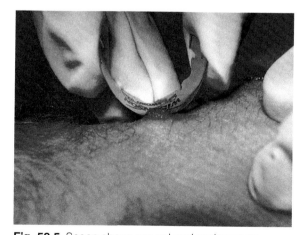

Fig. 58.5 Scoop shave around and under nevus.

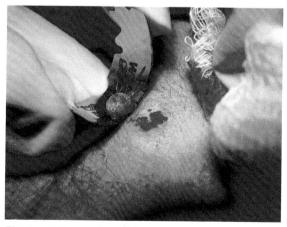

Fig. 58.6 Complete excision.

Razor Blade Excision for Shallow Basal Cell Carcinomas of the Nose

Rationale:

- Excision of even small tumors of the distal nose, to include the tip and alae nasi, can result in significant cosmetic defects that are difficult to repair.
- Basal cell carcinomas (BCCs) occur in a disproportionate frequency on the distal nose, which also represents a region at high risk for recurrence.
- Therefore, it is appropriate to perform Mohs micrographic surgery (MMS) on these small tumors in an attempt to completely eradicate the lesion but also take advantage of the tissue sparing inherent to the technique.
- Consequently, a technique to obtain very thin discs of tissue for examination by frozen section is presented.
- Because of extreme sharpness of the razor blade, very thin tissue specimens are attainable.
- If this initial section is negative for tumor, the wound may be allowed to heal by second intention with the expectation of excellent results.
- If the pilosebaceous units are preserved, they supply both the dermal bulk and the epithelial cells for epidermal regeneration.

Technique:

- After anesthetizing the area, the tumor is debulked with an appropriately sized curette.

- A 1–2 mm rim of normal-appearing tissue is then excised (*Fig. 59.1*).
- The razor blade is bowed slightly downward to adjust for depth.
- An assistant can supply stabilization and counter-traction with a cotton-tipped applicator (*Fig. 59.2*).
- If the specimen proves to be negative, the wound is allowed heal by granulation and epithelialization (*Figs 59.3 and 59.4*).

Advantages:

- A razor blade permits a thinner disc of tissue than a standard scalpel blade.
- Maximum amount of normal tissue is preserved.
- Shallow defect may not need sophisticated repair.
- Cost-effective if repair is avoided.

Caveat:

- If the tissue specimen contains residual tumor after the first excision, a standard scalpel should be used for subsequent stages as the advantage of the razor blade is lost.

Reference:

Grabski WJ, Salasche SJ. Razor blade excision of Mohs' specimens for superficial basal cell carcinomas of the distal nose. J Dermatol Surg Oncol 1988; 14:1290–1292.

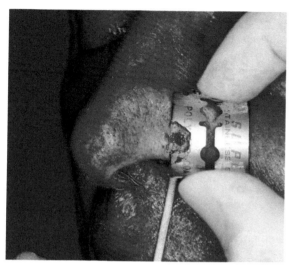

Fig. 59.1 Initiating excision after curettage of BCC. Note stabilizing CTA within nostril under ala nasi.

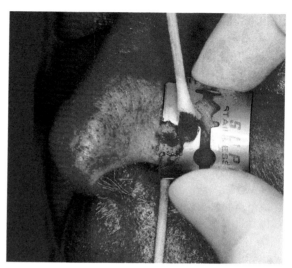

Fig. 59.2 Continuing excision using CTA for counter-traction.

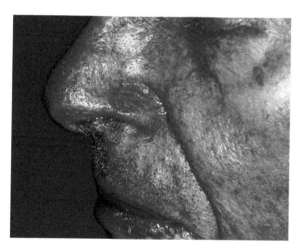

Fig. 59.3 Healing by second intention.

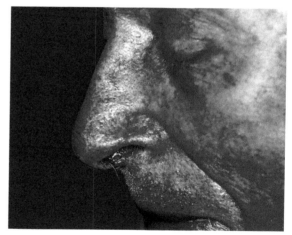

Fig. 59.4 Healing complete.

TIP 60
Alternate Use of Forceps
Freeze with a Squeeze

Rationale:

- There are several different modalities used to remove multiple skin tags from the neck, inframammary region, axilla or groin.
- Some patients prefer to tie the tags off with small string or hair until they necrose and subsequently drop off.
- Although this technique works, it can be quite painful and may take days before the tag falls off.
- Many surgeons use scissors to perform a snip excision.
- The use of liquid nitrogen is quite an effective modality for the removal of skin tags.
- However, using the standard Cry-Ac canister, the large spray zone beyond the tag increases the area of destruction, possibly leading to delayed healing, hypopigmentation or scarring.
- By using forceps, the area frozen can be restricted to a smaller area of just the tag itself.

Technique:

- Pour liquid nitrogen into a properly secured Styrofoam cup (*Fig. 60.1*).
- Some patients may not be able to tolerate the pain involved.
- In this case, either a topical anesthetic cream such as Elamax or EMLA may be used, or local infiltration with 1% lidocaine with epinephrine may be used at the base of each lesion to be frozen.
- Use a folded 4 × 4 gauze over the handle of the forceps to dip into the liquid nitrogen for about 10–15 seconds (*Fig. 60.1*).
- The forceps will be cold to the touch and frosted.
- The tag is then pinched between the frozen tips of the forceps for approximately 15 seconds (*Fig. 60.2*).
- Repeat this procedure for each of the tags.

Advantages:

- Decreases the pain associated with the cryotherapy of skin tags as well as decreasing the injury to surrounding, normal tissue.
- Insures a better cosmetic result.
- No bleeding associated with this procedure and bandaging not required.

Variation:

- A hemostat can be substituted for the forceps in this pearl (*Fig. 60.3*).

Reference:

Kuwahara RT, Huber JD, Ray SH. Surgical pearl: forceps method for freezing benign lesion. J Am Acad Dermatol 2000; 43:306–307.

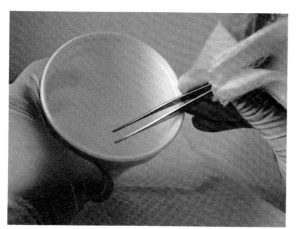

Fig. 60.1 Forceps dipped into Styrofoam cup with liquid nitrogen.

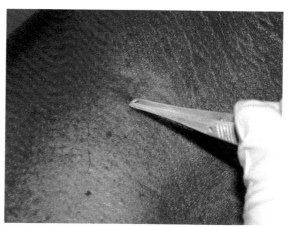

Fig. 60.2 Forceps applied to lesion, turning lesion white.

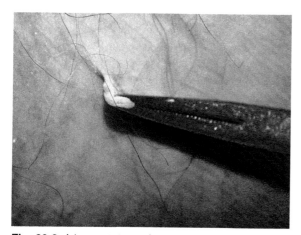

Fig. 60.3 A hemostat may be used instead of forceps.

TIP 61

Towel Clamp-Assisted Closure for Wounds under Significant Tension

 Rationale:

- Certain wounds, which are under high closure tension, may benefit from tissue expansion.
- There are several traditional surgical techniques available to achieve acute tissue expansion.
- A technique that does not require a period of delay or special expensive instrumentation would provide an alternative to achieve optimal wound closure.
- Taking advantage of the skin's regionally variable ability to 'creep,' towel clamps can be utilized to achieve some degree of immediate intraoperative tissue expansion.

 Technique:

- After undermining, each pointed end of a sterile towel clamp is inserted at least 1 cm from the wound edge and carried through the full thickness of skin and dermis (Figs 61.1, 61.2 and 61.3).
- This must be done far enough back from the edges of the wound to avoid tearing and pulling through the skin at the wound edge.
- The instrument is then clamped and may be left for up to 20 minutes to achieve significant tissue creep (Fig. 61.4).
- The instrument is then unclamped, often revealing sufficient expansion to achieve closure of large wounds now under significantly less tension.
- Buried sutures are placed to close off dead space, relieve residual tension and insure wound edge eversion (Fig. 61.5).

- Alternatively, sutures can be placed prior to clamping and then tied once the clamps are in place and stretch has occurred.
- Finally, the closure is completed in a routine manner (Fig. 61.6).

 Variants:

- For smaller defects, some stretch may be attained by placing a temporary large vertical or horizontal mattress suture across the area of highest tension.
- The wound is then closed inward toward the tension from the apices and the temporary mattress suture removed.

 Advantages:

- This is a simple and efficient technique which provides a high degree of tissue expansion.
- It is particularly useful for scalp defects.

 Caveat:

- Postoperative 'fang marks' may be present from the towel clamp stab wounds (Fig. 61.6).

 Reference:

Liu CM, McKenna J, Griess A. Surgical pearl: the use of towel clamps to re-approximate wound edges under tension. J Am Acad Dermatol 2004; 50:273–274.

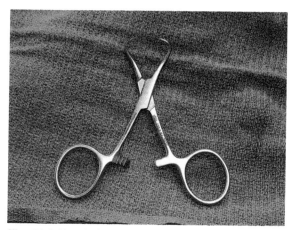

Fig. 61.1 Towel clamp.

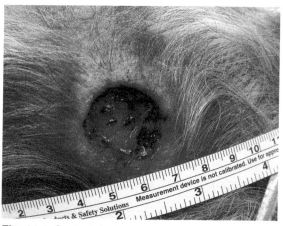

Fig. 61.2 Scalp defect.

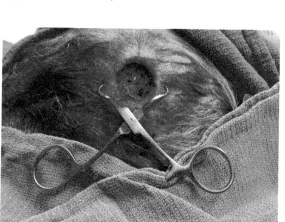

Fig. 61.3 Sterile towel clamp inserted into skin at point of greatest tension with entry points at least 1 cm back from the wound edge.

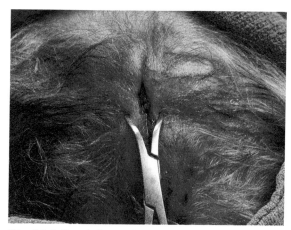

Fig. 61.4 Towel clamp closes the wound completely, where it will be left in place for up to 20 minutes.

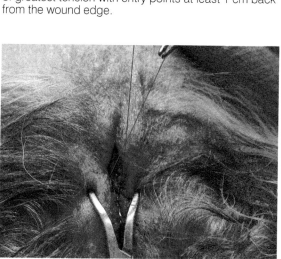

Fig. 61.5 Buried sutures placed before the towel clamp is closed.

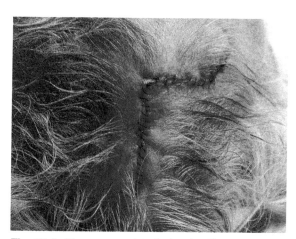

Fig. 61.6 Closure completed, showing 'fang marks' from the towel clamp teeth.

TIP 62
The Cotton-Tipped Applicator (CTA)
The Ever-Ready, Multipurpose Superstar

 Rationale:
- There are multiple and varied uses for the ubiquitous cotton-tipped applicator (CTA).
- The CTA is readily available and inexpensive.
- It is quite easy to include the CTA in a standard tray set-up or to individually package 10–15 CTAs to be sterilized and then added to the surgical tray if multiple applicators are needed.
- Some innovative uses of the CTA include turning the surgical light or electrocautery machine on when the surgeon is already gloved.
- The CTA can substitute as a finger and be used to apply pressure to insure hemostasis, counter-traction, stabilization or visualization during surgery.
- The main advantage is that, while acting as a finger proxy, the fingers are kept out of the surgical field.
- CTAs can also be used to apply antibacterial or Vaseline ointment to the wound after surgery.
- The CTA can substitute for various other instruments or devices such as a marking pen.
- They can also be used to apply liquid nitrogen to lesions close to the eyes.
- Adequate anesthesia can also be tested with the CTA.

 Technique:
- For hemostasis, roll a dry CTA back and forth over the operative field.
- This allows the surgeon to identify the bleeding vessel and lightly spot electrocoagulate the vessel (*Fig. 62.1*).
- To use as a marking pen, dip wooden handle into the blood of the wound and then use it to mark areas to be further excised or to design the repair (*Fig. 62.2*).
- For a finer line, snap the wooden portion and use the sharp point.

- In testing the adequacy of local anesthesia, break the wooden handle into two parts and use the sharp edge to poke skin and test sensation.
- For cryotherapy in delicate areas, pour liquid nitrogen (LN2) into Styrofoam cup, partially unwind the cotton of the CTA, twirl into a fine point, dip the CTA into the LN2 and apply directly to lesion to be removed.
- For stabilization of the nasal ala, have assistant place two CTAs into the nasal opening (*Fig. 62.3*).
- The non-dominant surgical hand can be used to apply stabilizing pressure to the nasal tip.
- This will flatten the nasal ala and allows for an even removal of tissue on the ala cutaneous surface.
- This same technique can also be used to stabilize the tissue when using a razor blade for excision of a thin disc of tissue (see Tip 58), when suturing a full thickness skin graft or when excising an ellipse (*Figs 62.4 and 62.5*).
- Spot counter-traction can be applied most anywhere (*Fig. 62.6*).

 Advantages:
- The CTA is inexpensive, disposable, versatile and easy to use.
- It is smaller and more expendable than a finger.
- It maintains a clearly visible surgical field by applying counter-traction, stabilization and hemostasis while minimizing the danger of accidental puncture wounds.

 Reference:
Orengo I, Salasche SJ. Surgical pearl: the cotton-tipped applicator – the ever-ready, multipurpose superstar. J Am Acad Dermatol 1994; 31:658–660.

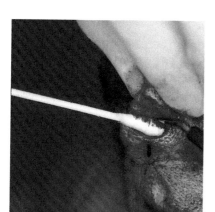

Fig. 62.1 A CTA rolled back and forth provides a clear view of focal bleeders for electrocoagulation.

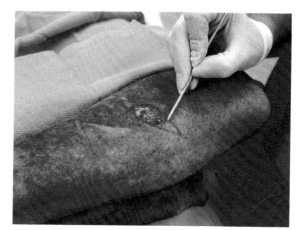

Fig. 62.2 A CTA as a marking pen.

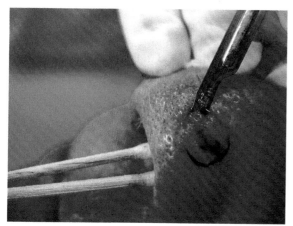

Fig. 62.3 Nasal ala stabilized for excision.

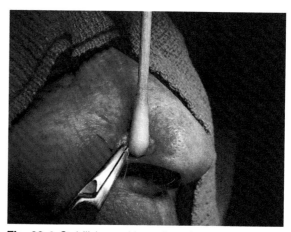

Fig. 62.4 Stabilizing a skin graft on the nasal ala while suturing.

Fig. 62.5 Applying counter-traction for elliptical excision.

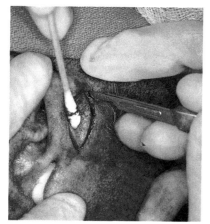

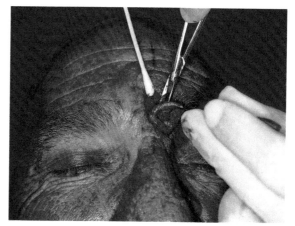

Fig. 62.6 Counter-traction.

TIP 63
The Tongue Depressor
More Than Say 'Ah'

 Rationale:

- It is difficult to immobilize free margins such as ear lobes and lips.
- The tongue depressor is an excellent tool to stabilize the free margins during procedures such as split ear lobe or cleft ear lobe repairs.
- Tissue tends to adhere to the wood.
- The tongue depressor can also be used to stabilize a punch biopsy specimen that needs to be halved or for procuring single hairs for hair transplantation.

 Technique:

Ear lobe repair:
- With the non-dominant hand, the surgeon should place a sterile tongue depressor blade posterior to the ear lobe to stabilize the patient's ear lobe during repair (*Fig. 63.1*).
- This allows the surgeon to accurately excise the tissue with little movement of the ear lobe.
- It also decreases the potential for an accidental sharp injury to the surgeon or the assistant.

Punch biopsy:
- When dividing a punch biopsy specimen for histology and culture or for immunofluorescence, place biopsy epidermal side up on sterile tongue depressor.
- Then stabilize with a forceps and divide with a 15 blade (*Fig. 63.2*).

Hair transplantation:
- This technique can be easily applied for hair transplant specimens where the surgeon is trying to get one or two hairs per graft.
- An ellipse of hair-bearing tissue is excised from the posterior scalp.
- This tissue is then placed on the tongue depressor and individual hair bulbs are easily excised on this stable surface (*Fig. 63.3*).

 Advantages:

- The tongue depressor allows the surgeon to have an inexpensive, disposable, stable support for surgery involving free margins or free tissue.
- As an added benefit, it also protects the surgeon against needlesticks or sharp injuries during the procedure.
- An additional advantage is that the wet tissue adheres to the wood of the tongue depressor, increasing the stability of the small biopsy material.

 References:

Inman VD, Pariser RJ. Biopsy technique pearl: obtaining an optimal split punch-biopsy specimen. J Am Acad Dermatol 2003; 48:273–274.

Smith C, Glasser DA. Surgical pearl: repair of split or deformed ear lobe with a tongue depressor for stabilization during surgery. J Am Acad Dermatol 1998; 38:990–991.

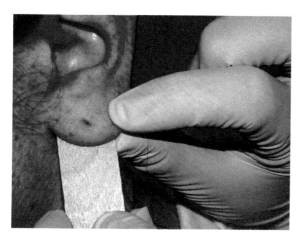

Fig. 63.1 Tongue depressor behind ear lobe.

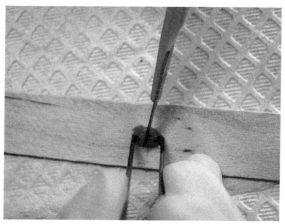

Fig. 63.2 Biopsy specimen being bisected on tongue depressor.

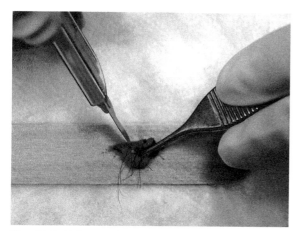

Fig. 63.3 Hair transplantation ellipse with single hairs being dissected.

TIP 64
The Universal Paper Clip
There's Always One in the Desk Drawer

Rationale:

- Some patients many present with many comedones, milia, small cysts or syringomas that they want removed.
- A quick, easy and inexpensive instrument that can be used to remove them is a paper clip.
- The paper clip is a substitute for the more expensive comedo extractors that are commercially available.

Technique:

- For all of these lesions, after cleaning the skin with an alcohol wipe, use a #11 blade to puncture or open up the lesion (*Fig. 64.1*).
- No anesthesia is required.
- Then use the open end of a paper clip to apply firm pressure in parallel fashion to the lesion popping it out (*Fig. 64.2*).
- The paper clip should be an unused, right out of the clip box, and cleaned with an alcohol wipe prior to use.

Advantages:

- The use of the paper clip in the removal of comedones, milia, small cysts and syringomas is inexpensive and easy.
- The paper clip is disposable.
- There are various sizes of paper clips that may be used.
- A medium-sized paper clip (ARCO #1) is the most universal and convenient.
- There is no need for re-sterilization since this 'instrument' is inexpensive and disposable.

Reference:

Cvancara JL, Meffert JJ. Surgical pearl: versatile paper clip comedone extractor for acne surgery. J Am Acad Dermatol 1999; 40:477–478.

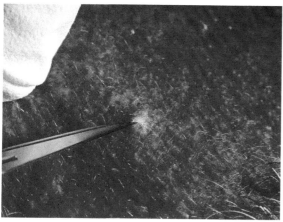

Fig. 64.1 Use a #11 blade to puncture the top of the milium.

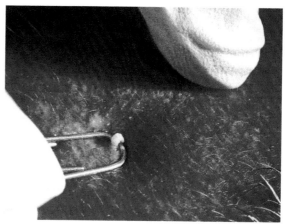

Fig. 64.2 Downward pressure initiates expression of contents and most of cyst contents are removed.

TIP 65
The Hyfrecator
Low-Tech, Yet Efficient

 Rationale:

- Selected, small benign lesions do not require high-tech instruments, such as lasers, for removal.
- The Hyfrecator, an instrument ubiquitously present in any cutaneous surgeon's office, easily treats a variety of small benign lesions including sebaceous hyperplasia, skin tags, telangiectasis, flat warts, fibrous papules, molluscum contagiosum and dermatosis papulosa nigra (DPN) (*Fig. 65.1*).

 Technique:

- Depending on patient desire or pain tolerance, either a topical anesthetic cream such as Elamax or EMLA may be used or local infiltration with 1% lidocaine with epinephrine may be used at the base of each lesion.
- For skin tags, flat warts, sebaceous hyperplasia, fibrous papules, molluscum and DPN, the Hyfrecator is tuned to the lowest possible setting.
- It is permissible to use any of the fine pointed tips (*Fig. 65.2*).
- Gently apply the Hyfrecator tip directly to the lesion surface and initiate current flow until the lesion melts away or necroses (*Fig. 65.3*).
- The damaged tissue can be blotted away with a gauze sponge (*Figs 65.4 and 65.5*).
- Healing is rapid with only minimal cleansing and hydrating ointment.

 Advantages:

- The Hyfrecator is a cost-effective method for removing small lesions.
- The low-tech procedure is accompanied by little discomfort to the patient, yet provides effective ablation of the lesion.
- There is minimal scarring associated with this technique, and multiple lesions can be treated at one sitting.

 Caveats:

- Make sure any alcohol used to cleanse the area has evaporated: otherwise, it could ignite.
- Make sure that if the patient is on oxygen it is turned off as oxygen is flammable and the spark of the Hyfrecator could ignite the oxygen.

 Reference:

Bader RS, Scarborough DA. Surgical pearl: intralesional electrodessication of sebaceous hyperplasia. J Am Acad Dermatol 2000; 42:127–128.

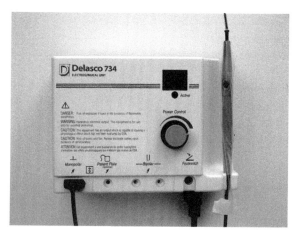

Fig. 65.1 Hyfrecator.

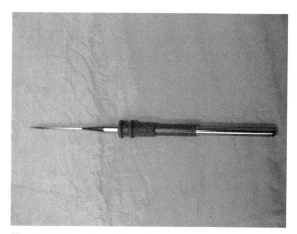

Fig. 65.2 Fine-tipped needle.

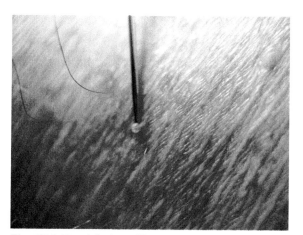

Fig. 65.3 Touch lesion with needle tip.

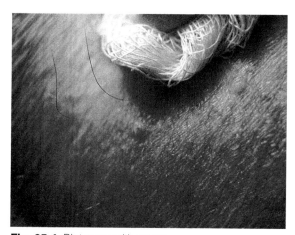

Fig. 65.4 Blot away with gauze.

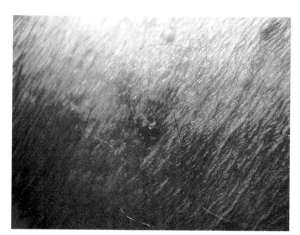

Fig. 65.5 Immediately postoperative.

The Punch Used as a Curette

Rationale:

- At times, the surgeon may not have a curette readily available for tumor debulking, curettage and desiccation, or for the removal of benign lesions.
- This typically occurs in charity clinics, nursing homes and ward consultations.
- However, disposable punch biopsy tools are available in most dermatology offices and are carried in the dermatologist's travel bag.
- They can substitute for a curette.
- Standard reusable curettes become dull with time and usually need to be sent out to be sharpened.
- Disposable curettes have the advantage of always being sharp since they have a one-time use.
- However, the expense ranging from $1 to $3 may be a disadvantage, especially for incidental functions.
- In selected situations, the disposable punch biopsy can be substituted for the curette and can be quite effective.

Technique:

- The surgeon should hold the punch biopsy instrument like a pencil (*Fig. 66.1*), mimicking the cutting angle of a standard curette.
- It is then used to scrape with the same pressure as with a standard curette (*Fig. 66.2*).

Advantages:

- The punch is inexpensive, sharp and disposable.
- The circular cutting edge is similar to that of a disposable curette.
- The instrument is readily available in all dermatology office practices.

Variation:

- The scalpel blade or razor blade edge can also be used as a curette to refine edges after shaving of a seborrheic keratosis or intradermal nevus.

Reference:

Quan LT, Orengo I. Surgical pearl: curetting with a punch. J Am Acad Dermatol 2000; 43:854–855.

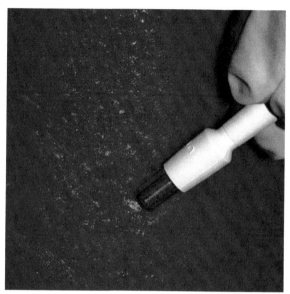

Fig. 66.1 Punch biopsy being held as a curette.

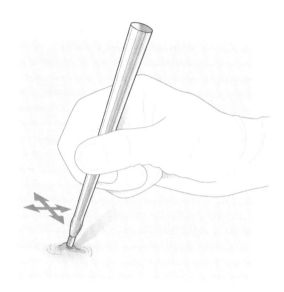

Fig. 66.2 The motion in which the disposable punch is used to mimic the curette.

Section 8

Nail

Rationale:

- Biopsy specimens of the nail matrix and bed are prone to both misorientation and crush distortion.
- Both may result in inadequate histologic interpretation.
- As securing a nail unit biopsy is difficult and time-consuming, every effort should be made to obtain the best possible specimen.
- The matrix and nail bed are comprised of their respective epithelial tissue and supporting dermis.
- There is no subcutaneous fat layer and the dermis is bound to the underlying periosteum of the distal phalanx (*Fig. 67.1*).
- Cutting and separation of the undersurface of the biopsy is therefore difficult without rough manipulation of the tissue.
- Also, as there is no fat to identify 'up or down,' properly orienting the tissue during blocking by the pathologist is problematic.

Technique:

- After avulsion of the nail plate and adequate exposure, the biopsy site is marked with an indelible surgical marker (*Fig. 67.2*).
- This effectively marks the epithelial surface even after tissue is placed in formalin.
- In the nail bed, the recommended orientation is longitudinal (*Fig. 67.3*).
- In the nail matrix, transverse or arced as distally as possible have been recommended (*Fig. 67.3*).
- However, there are situations (pigmented streaks, rapidly progressive scarring disease), where proximal and longitudinally oriented nail matrix biopsies are necessary.
- If possible, limit the width of the biopsy to 3 mm so that the defect can be closed by undermining at the periosteal level and sutured.

- Incisions with a scalpel or punch are made vertically down to the periosteum of the underlying bone.
- Separation is achieved by cutting all around the undersurface with a scalpel or curved sharp scissors.
- While doing this, the tissue may be secured and immobilized with gentle use of small, toothed forceps (*Fig. 67.4*).
- Alternatively, the specimen can be skewered through the dermis with the 30-gauge anesthetic needle (*Figs 67.4 and 67.5*).
- After passing it through the tissue, bend the tip with the needle holder, so the specimen is not lost when lifted off (*Fig. 67.5*).
- The separated specimen with the colored epithelial surface is ready to be placed in the specimen jar (*Fig. 67.6*).

Advantages:

- Avulsing nail plate allows direct visualization of where to biopsy.
- Avoids misorienting tissue; epithelial surface critical for histologic diagnosis.
- Avoids crush or squeeze injury that may interfere with tissue orientation.

Variant:

- Some surgeons prefer to punch through the intact nail plate.
- Soak the nail in warm water for 15 minutes prior to the biopsy to soften the nail.

References:

Rich P. Nail biopsy: indications and methods. J Dermatol Surg Oncol 1992; 18:673.

Salasche SJ. Surgery. In: Scher RK, Daniel CR III, eds. Nails: therapy, diagnosis, surgery. Philadelphia: WB Saunders; 1997:326–340.

Scher RK. Biopsy of the matrix of the nail. J Dermatol Surg Oncol 1980; 16:19.

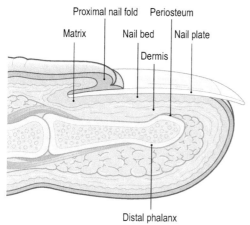

Fig. 67.1 Diagram of nail unit: no subcutaneous fat in nail unit.

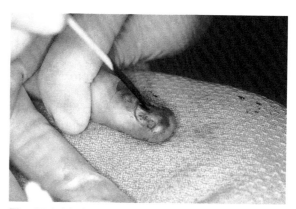

Fig. 67.2 Marking the biopsy site with gentian violet.

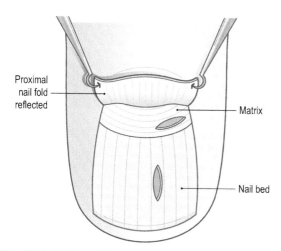

Fig. 67.3 Preferred biopsy orientation on nail unit.

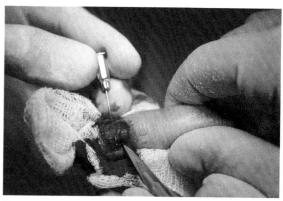

Fig. 67.4 After incising to periosteum, tissue secured with needle.

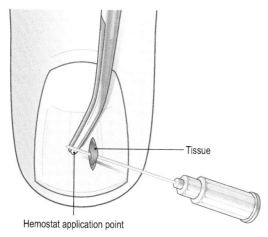

Fig. 67.5 Use hemostat to bend needle tip and prevent loss of specimen.

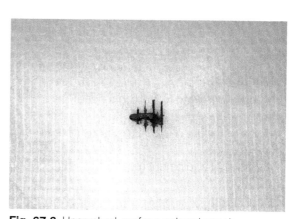

Fig. 67.6 Uncrushed, surface-colored specimen.

Nail Matrix Exploration and Retraction Suture for Exposure of the Proximal Nail Groove

Rationale:

- Exposure of the nail matrix is required for it to be examined and biopsied.
- This is achieved by reflecting the proximal nail fold.
- This procedure is known as the 'nail matrix exploration.'
- Procedures in this confined space of the proximal nail groove (which has the nail matrix as its floor) require sustained clear visualization.
- Also, instruments like skin hooks and forceps may crush or tear the nail fold tissue.

Technique:

- The exploration is initiated by making bilateral, tangential relaxing incisions at the junction of the proximal and lateral nail folds (*Fig. 68.1*).
- These are full-thickness incisions and should extend from the free edge to the proximal limit of the underlying proximal nail groove.
- Insertion of a Freer septum elevator precludes cutting down into matrix tissue (*Fig. 68.2*).
- Reflection of the proximal nail fold reveals the matrix area (*Fig. 68.3*).
- Retraction stitches, may be any non-absorbable suture such as inexpensive 4-0 or 5-0-nylon (*Fig. 68.4*).
- Paired sutures are placed back about 3 mm back from the edge of the proximal nail fold and about 5 mm apart.
- The insertion point of the needle is upward through the undersurface of the proximal nail fold.
- Both sutures are kept long, so they may be held and retracted at a distance from the operative site (*Fig. 68.4*).
- Skin hooks may be used but are less flexible and may damage tissue (*Fig. 68.5*).
- At the end of the procedure, the fold is replaced to its normal anatomic position and either sutured or steri-stripped into place (*Fig. 68.6*).

Advantages:

- Keeps unneeded instruments out of the small, confined surgical field.
- Does not injure or crush the tissue of the proximal nail fold.
- Inexpensive.
- No special equipment required.

References:

Rich PS, Nail surgery. In: Bolognia JL, Jorizzo JL, Rapini RP, eds. Dermatology. London: Elsevier; 2003:2321–2330.

Salasche SJ, Orengo I. Surgical pearl: the retraction suture. J Am Acad Dermatol 1994; 30:118–120.

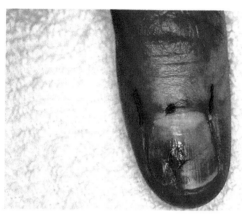

Fig. 68.1 Proposed lines of incision for nail matrix exploration. Split nail following blunt trauma. (From Salasche SJ. Surgery. In: Scher RK, Daniel CR III. Nails: Therapy, Diagnosis, Surgery. WB Saunders, Philadelphia. 1977.)

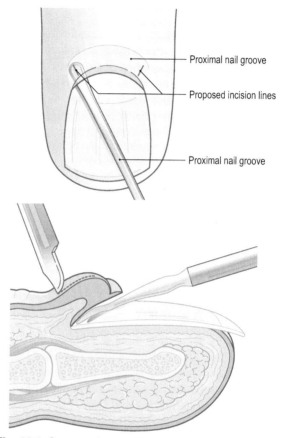

- Proximal nail groove
- Proposed incision lines
- Proximal nail groove

Fig. 68.2 Septum elevator in groove allows incision of fold with no danger of causing matrix injury.

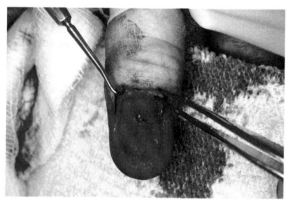

Fig. 68.3 Proximal nail fold reflected, revealing injury. (From Salasche SJ. Surgery. In: Scher RK, Daniel CR III. Nails: Therapy, Diagnosis, Surgery. WB Saunders, Philadelphia. 1977.)

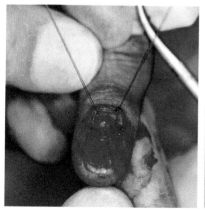

Fig. 68.4 Retraction sutures reveal acquired digital fibrokeratoma overlying matrix. (From Salasche SJ, Orengo I. Surgical pearl: the retraction suture. J Am Acad Dermatol 1994; 30:118–120.)

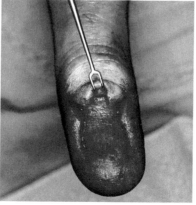

Fig. 68.5 Skin hook reflects, but digs into tissue. (From Salasche SJ. Surgery. In: Scher RK, Daniel CR III. Nails: Therapy, Diagnosis, Surgery. WB Saunders, Philadelphia. 1977.)

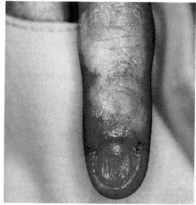

Fig. 68.6 Simple interrupted stitches placed to complete procedure.

Rationale:

- In the postoperative period, patients require bulky, compressive dressings for comfort, to prevent edema and to aid in hemostasis.
- Even routine bumping into objects can be excruciatingly painful.
- Dressings should secure the non-adherent wound covering, but have enough expansive 'give' to allow normal swelling and edema without constriction.
- They should be easy to change by the patient at home.

Technique:

- At the completion of surgery, the surgical site is covered with a thin layer of petrolatum-based or ointment and a non-adherent pad such as a Telfa or Release Pad (*Figs 69.1 and 69.2*).
- This can be secured with paper tape but not in a completely circumferential manner as this might prove constrictive.
- Some layered loose gauze will add bulk and absorbency to the dressing (*Fig. 69.3*).
- Finally, several overlapping layers of X-Span or Surgitube are used to secure the inner layers and add compressive bulk (*Figs 69.4, 69.5 and 69.6*).

- No special instruments or devices are needed for layering. Just twist the dressing a half turn and fit another layer over the digit.
- Dressings should be changed on a daily basis.

Advantages:

- Dressing is comfortable, compressive, absorbent and shields against trauma.
- Easy-to-use dressing materials.
- Easy to learn and perform by patients or their family.

Variant:

- Other tube dressings are commercially available and may be substituted if they have the same qualities as the X-Span.

Reference:

Salasche SJ. Surgery. In: Scher RK, Daniel CR III, eds. Nails: therapy, diagnosis, surgery. Philadelphia: WB Saunders; 1997:326–349.

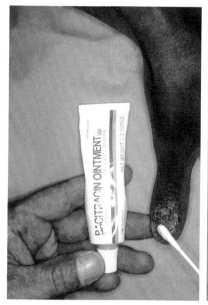

Fig. 69.1 Application of antibiotic ointment.

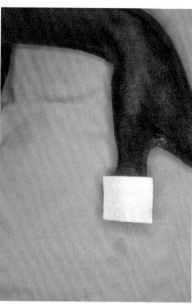

Fig. 69.2 Covered with non-adherent dressing.

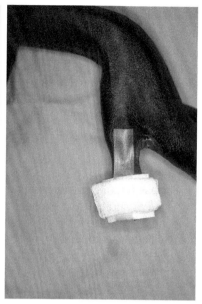

Fig. 69.3 Bulky gauze layer.

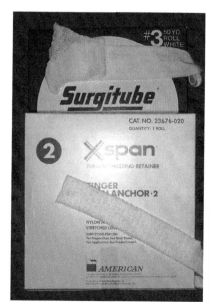

Fig. 69.4 Compressive tubular dressings.

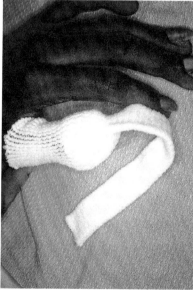

Fig. 69.5 Initial layer of tubular gauze.

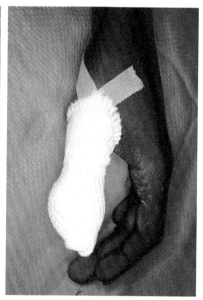

Fig. 69.6 Double layer secured.

Rationale:

- For many cutaneous surgical procedures, antiseptic preparation and sterile isolation of the surgical site is mandatory to prevent infection.
- Isolating and draping individual fingers and toes can be cumbersome.
- An ideal method is having the patient put on a sterile surgical glove.

Technique:

- Choose a glove size larger than the patient would normally wear.
- As a learning trial and experience, use the opposite hand glove, invert it and have the patient practice having it put on using the usual sterile technique.
- After antiseptically prepping the area, the patient is assisted in putting on the surgical glove as if he or she were to be part of the surgical team (*Fig. 70.1*).
- After this has been accomplished, the tip of the glove finger is pulled down and snipped off of the appropriate glove (*Fig. 70.2*).
- Be sure to pull the tip of the glove away from the finger so the finger is not inadvertently injured.
- This allows the glove to be pulled back on itself proximally to adequately expose the surgical site (*Fig. 70.3)* prior to performing the procedure (*Fig. 70.4*).

Advantage:

- This offers a relatively easy method of designing and maintaining a sterile field for nail unit surgery.

Variants:

- An exsanguinating tourniquet can be fashioned by tightly rolling the snipped glove finger backward instead of just draping it back loosely.
- Caution should be exercised in doing this as usually the tourniquet is applied only during the part of the procedure when bleeding may occur.
- If there is much preparation time prior to cutting, the tourniquet may be left in place too long.

Reference:

Salasche SJ. Surgery. In: Scher RK, Daniel CR III, eds. Nails: therapy, diagnosis, surgery. Philadelphia: WB Saunders; 1997:326–340.

Siegle RJ, Swanson NA. Nail Surgery: a review. J Dermatol Surg Oncol 1982:659–666.

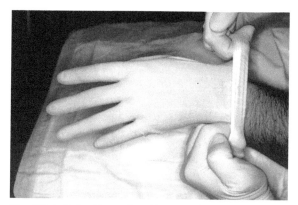

Fig. 70.1 Patient is assisted into sterile glove.

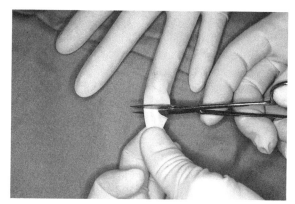

Fig. 70.2 Finger of glove pulled away from finger and snipped off.

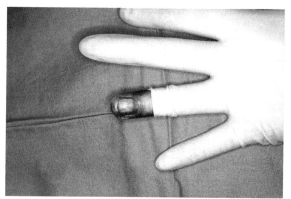

Fig. 70.3 Glove rolled back to expose sterile operating field.

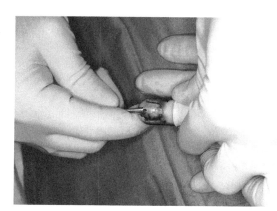

Fig. 70.4 Procedure performed.

The Proximal Nail Plate Avulsion

Rationale:

- Technically, a distal avulsions is easier to perform.
- However, occasionally there is no free edge to the nail plate, making distal avulsion difficult (*Fig. 71.1*).
- This may occur with onychomycosis, prior avulsions, infection and other conditions.

Technique:

- After anesthesia and prepping of the surgical area, the septum elevator or another similar instrument is introduced under the proximal nail fold into the far end of the proximal nail groove (*Fig. 71.2*).
- At this point the elevator handle is rotated from distal to proximal (*Fig. 71.3*).
- If done correctly, the elevator slips under the most proximal portion of the newly forming nail plate (*Fig. 71.4*).
- It can then be advanced distally between the nail plate and bed until it comes out distally (*Fig. 71.5*).
- Care must be taken to also exert some force upward against the undersurface of the plate in order not to damage the matrix or bed as the instrument is advanced distally.
- Once the elevator is exposed, simply lifting upward results in separation of the entire nail plate (*Fig. 71.6*).

Advantages:

- This works well for situations when nail avulsion is required, but there is not a clearly defined free edge to the nail plate to perform the more standard distal avulsion.
- This technique is based on the loose attachment of the newly forming nail plate over the matrix area.
- This loose attachment accounts for the white color of the lunula.
- It is actually an air space between the newly formed nail and the highly vascularized matrix.
- The matrix is actually quite reddish in appearance when the plate is removed.

References:

Daniel CR III. Basic nail plate avulsion. J Dermatol Surg Oncol 1992; 18:685.
Scher RK. Surgical avulsion of nail plates by a proximal to distal technique. J Dermatol Surg Oncol 1981; 7:296.

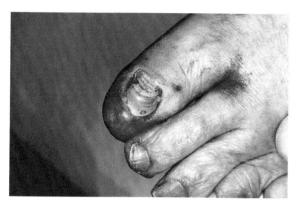

Fig. 71.1 Dystrophic nail without distal free edge.

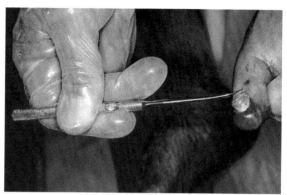

Fig. 71.2 Septum elevator introduced into proximal nail groove. (From Salasche SJ. Surgery. In: Scher RK, Daniel CR III. Nails: Therapy, Diagnosis, Surgery. Philadelphia, WB Saunders.)

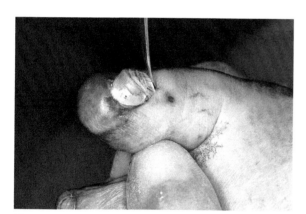

Fig. 71.3 Elevator is rotated proximally.

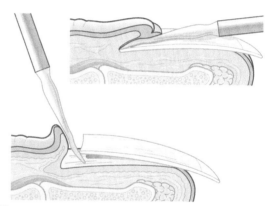

Fig. 71.4 Rotation brings elevator under newly forming nail plate above matrix.

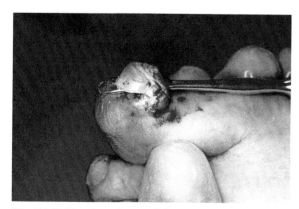

Fig. 71.5 Elevator advanced distally while exerting upward pressure on undersurface of nail plate. (From Salasche SJ. Surgery. In: Scher RK, Daniel CR III. Nails: Therapy, Diagnosis, Surgery. Philadelphia, WB Saunders 1997.)

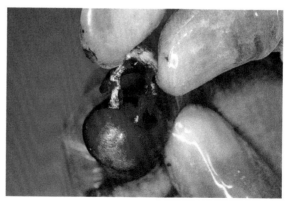

Fig. 71.6 Nail almost avulsed.

TIP 72

Postphenol Matricectomy Injection to Prolong Anesthesia and Prevent Lymphangitis

Rationale:

- Partial or complete matricectomy can be done with full-strength 88% phenol.
- Phenol acts by denaturing protein of the matrix epithelial cells.
- Tissue is destroyed to the mid-dermal level and heals by scar formation.
- There is usually intense pain for the first 24 hours following phenol matricectomy.
- A chemical lymphangitis often occurs after the first 24 hours.
- Injecting a short-acting corticosteroid and a long-acting anesthetic during the immediate postoperative period can prevent both of these sequelae.

Technique:

- A mixture consisting of 0.4 cc dexamethasone and 0.6 cc bupivacaine is drawn up in a single syringe (*Fig. 72.1*).
- Small amounts (0.2–0.3 cc) of this mixture are injected into several sites along the proximal nail fold (*Fig. 72.2*).
- This will give the patient sustained anesthesia for about 12 hours and prevent the chemically induced lymphangitis.

Advantage:

- This simple maneuver eliminates two of the most bothersome side effects of chemical matricectomy.

Caveat:

- As with any injection into a constricted site, small amounts will avoid tamponade pressure problems.

Reference:

Salasche SJ, Peters V. Tips on nail surgery. Cutis 1984; 35:428.

Siegle RJ, Harkness JJ, Swanson NA. The phenol alcohol technique for permanent matricectomy. Arch Derm. 1984:348–350.

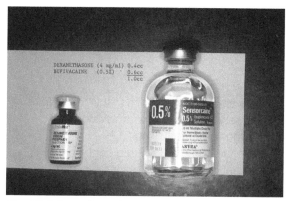

Fig. 72.1 Ingredients for postoperative injection.

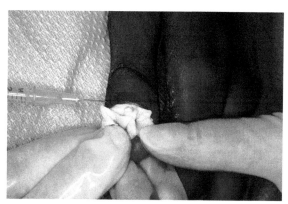

Fig. 72.2 One injection site along proximal nail fold.

Decompression of a Subungual Hematoma

Rationale:

- Crush injuries to the nail unit may cause painful subungual hematoma.
- Blood collects between the nail matrix/bed and the overlying nail plate (*Figs 73.1 and 73.2*).
- As the attachment between the matrix and the overlying nail plate is considerably looser than the bed/plate attachment, blood usually collects there.
- Pain is severe and throbbing and may last for days, interfering with sleep, walking or use of the affected hand.
- Discoloration that progresses from blue to yellowish-purple during resolution can be unsightly and last for months.
- Decompression offers immediate relief from pain and tenderness.

Technique:

- The time-tested method is decompression with a heated paper clip.
- One end of the clip is heated to red-hot in an open flame.
- It is then allowed to cool so no longer glowing but, while still very hot, pressed gently into the nail plate (*Fig. 73.3*).
- The heated clip easily melts through the nail plate allowing hematoma fluid to ooze out. Gentle compression aids complete evacuation (*Fig. 73.4*).
- No anesthesia is required.
- The hole bored by the procedure must grow out with the nail plate.
- If its edges get ragged, they can be filed or covered with an adhesive.

Advantages:

- Inexpensive; no special equipment needed.
- Easy to perform.

Variants:

- There are several variants to this technique; most require some decompression and anesthesia of the nail unit.
- These include boring with a dental drill, using a nail trephine, boring with a large-bore needle or a # 11 surgical blade.
- Trephine with a disposable electrocautery.
- The CO_2 laser without anesthesia (with settings of 20 W, 1 mm focussed spot) will, with several pulses, melt through the plate.

References:

Helms A, Brodell RT. Surgical pearl: prompt treatment of subungual hematoma by decompression. J Am Acad Dermatol 2000; 42:508–509.

Meek S, White M. Subungual hematomas; is simple trephining enough? J Acad Emerg Med 1998; 15:269–271.

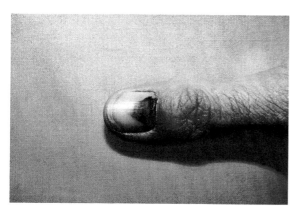

Fig. 73.1 Subungual hematoma over nail matrix after 1 month.

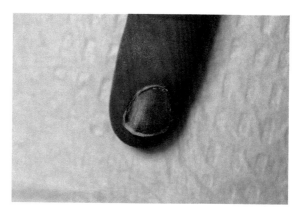

Fig. 73.2 Subungual hematoma over nail bed and matrix. (Courtesy, Robert Brodell, MD.)

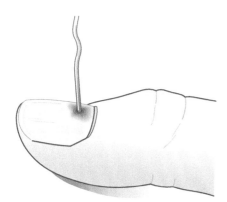

Fig. 73.3 Decompression with heated paper clip.

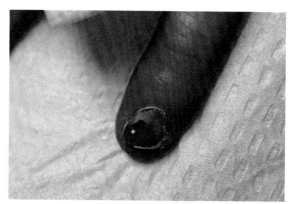

Fig. 73.4 Evacuation of hematoma. (Courtesy, Robert Brodell, MD.)

Section 9

Regional tips

Pinwheel Flap and Direct Galeotomy to Close Circular Defects on the Scalp

Rationale:

- Non-melanoma skin cancers occur not infrequently on the vertex of the scalp where partial baldness allows excessive ultraviolet radiation exposure.
- There is not much recruitable extra skin on the scalp.
- On the scalp, pinwheel flaps accomplish the same goal as the Mercedes flap but the type of tissue transfer is with rotational movement, not advancement.

Technique

- Two or three rotation flaps are incised full thickness to include the galea aponeurotica.
- Each flap is cut with equal width and equal distance around the defect (*Fig. 74.1*).
- The flaps are rotated in succession toward the center of the defect and secured in standard fashion (*Figs 74.2 and 74.3*).
- When closure is under tension, additional rotation flaps can be added to the pinwheel or a direct galeotomy can expand the tissue.
- With the scalp flap raised and the galea exposed, a series of incisions just through the galea parallel with the advancing edge of the flap are made to minimize the constraint on advancement that this thick fascial band presents (*Figs 74.4, 74.5 and 74.6*).
- Criss-cross incisions can be made to further 'mesh' the galea, thus gaining even greater stretch.

Advantage:

- These flaps are very useful where the skin is thick, such as on the scalp and trunk where purse-string closures are not as useful.

Caveat:

- When performing direct galeotomy, be sure not to cut large vessels that lie directly above the galea aponeurotica in the lower, subcutaneous fat.

References:

Tromovitch TA, Stegman SJ, Glogau RG, eds. Flaps and grafts in dermatologic surgery. Lesions of the scalp. Chicago: Year Book Medical Publishers Inc.; 1989:73–82

Vecchione TR, Griffith L. Closure of scalp defects by using multiple flaps in a pinwheel design. Plast Reconstr Surg 1978; 62:74.

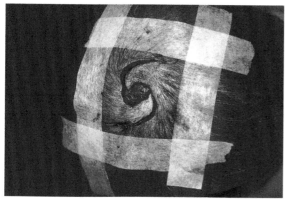

Fig. 74.1 Circular defect of vertex with pinwheel
closure. (From Salasche SJ, Bernstein G, Senkarik M.
Surgical Anatomy of the Skin. Norwalk, Appelton &
Lange, 1988.)

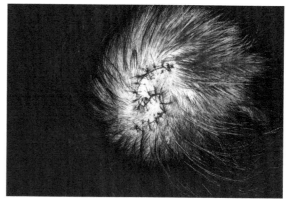

Fig. 74.2 Bilateral rotation flaps closed. (From
Salasche SJ, Bernstein G, Senkarik M. Surgical
Anatomy of the Skin. Norwalk, Appelton & Lange,
1988.)

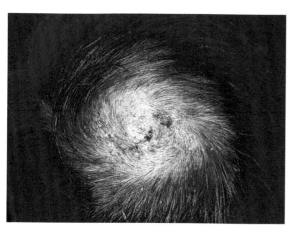

Fig. 74.3 Short-term healing.

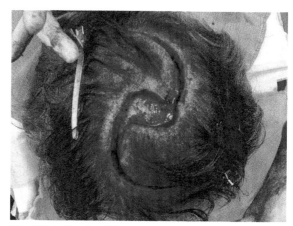

Fig. 74.4 Pinwheel flap requiring additional tissue
movement.

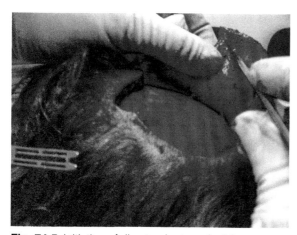

Fig. 74.5 Initiation of direct galeotomy incision.

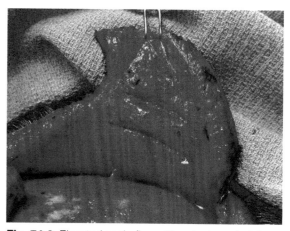

Fig. 74.6 Elevated scalp flap with galeotomy incisions
parallel to advancing edge.

Rationale:
- Surgery of the scalp poses unique problems.
- Hair creates several challenges: foremost, it may block precise excision and also get in the way of suture placement.
- Postoperative dressing is difficult to fashion and secure.
- Patients are not happy with extensive hair cutting, but will understand removal of a reasonable amount if it is explained why it is necessary.

Technique:
- Depending on lesion size and location as well as the intended repair, a sufficient amount of hair is clipped to insure good visualization and room to place sutures (*Fig. 75.1*).
- This is best done with a scissors.
- While a closer cut can be obtained with a razor blade, it is felt that the resulting nicks of the skin may increase the risk of bacterial colonization and subsequent infection (*Fig. 75.2*).
- Further control of unruly hair can be obtained by wetting with sterile saline or Hibiclens (chlorhexidine) scrubbing solution (*Fig. 75.3*).
- Other suggestions include the application of mousse gel, antibiotic ointments or barrettes.
- Probably the most efficient aide to keep hair out of the field is to combine one of the above with X-Span expandable mesh gauze.
- These come in various sizes for different body parts with the size indication marked on the box (*Fig. 75.4*).
- The advantage of this product is its elastic property that allows for a snug fit (*Fig. 75.5*).
- Once placed on the scalp, sufficient holes are snipped to allow an adequate surgical field, but small enough to hold the hair down (*Fig. 75.6*).
- If the hair becomes unruly while suturing, one way to keep it from entangling within the knot is to enlist an assistant.
- The assistant can hold the short free end of the suture up with an untoothed forceps so the surgeon can grasp it with the needle holder (*Figs 75.7 and 75.8*).

- This is repeated after each throw.
- The key is to have the assistant secure the free end immediately before it becomes woven into the loose hair.

 Advantage:
- All these maneuvers, if thought out pre-emptively, make scalp surgery easier.

 Caveats:
- None.

 Reference:
Salasche SJ. Surgical pearl: tips for scalp surgery. J Am Acad Dermatol 1994; 31:791–792.

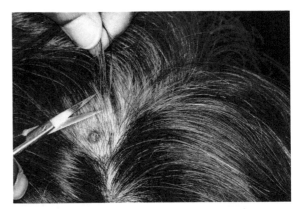

Fig. 75.1 Trimming hair. (From Salasche SJ. Surgical pearl: tips for scalp surgery. J Am Acad Dermatol 1994; 31:791–792.)

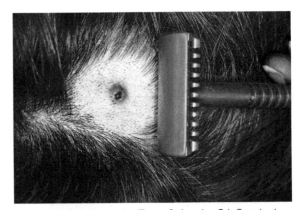

Fig. 75.2 Shaving hair. (From Salasche SJ. Surgical pearl: tips for scalp surgery. J Am Acad Dermatol 1994; 31:791–792.)

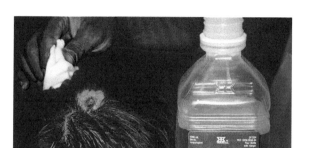

Fig. 75.3 Wetting hair with saline. (From Salasche SJ. Surgical pearl: tips for scalp surgery. J Am Acad Dermatol 1994; 31:791–792.)

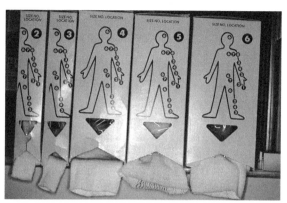

Fig. 75.4 Various sizes of X-Span. (From Salasche SJ. Surgical pearl: tips for scalp surgery. J Am Acad Dermatol 1994; 31:791–792.)

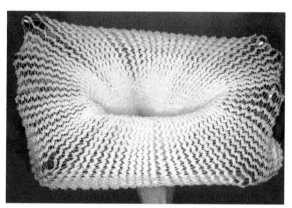

Fig. 75.5 Expandable material fits snuggly on scalp. (From Salasche SJ. Surgical pearl: tips for scalp surgery. J Am Acad Dermatol 1994; 31:791–792.)

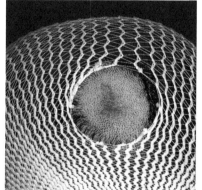

Fig. 75.6 X-Span in place with hole cut to expose surgical field. (From Salasche SJ. Surgical pearl: tips for scalp surgery. J Am Acad Dermatol 1994; 31:791–792.)

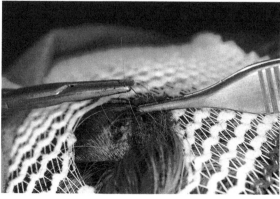

Fig. 75.7 Free end of suture held up for surgeon. (From Salasche SJ. Surgical pearl: tips for scalp surgery. J Am Acad Dermatol 1994; 31:791–792.)

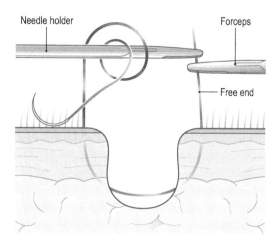

Fig. 75.8 Free end of suture held up for surgeon.

Rationale:

- Dressings for scalp wounds are difficult to fashion.
- The hair precludes securing them with standard adhesives.
- In order to be sufficiently compressive and support hemostasis, they need to be large and bulky (*Fig. 76.1*).
- These are uncomfortable and often come off at night in bed.
- It may be better to have a simple dressing that protects the wound from the environment, but requires no care.

 Technique:

- The key to this dressing is meticulous hemostasis.
- This should include 5 minutes of direct pressure after seemingly adequate hemostasis is attained.
- The wound and surrounding skin is covered by a layer of collodion (Collodion, Flexible, USP) (*Fig. 76.2*).
- This liquid is drizzled onto the wound with a cotton-tipped applicator.
- As it dries, it becomes a slightly opaque, whitish film (*Fig. 76.3*).
- Several successively applied layers may be required.
- This coating then acts as a protective seal (*Figs 76.3 and 76.4*).
- The film requires no care and remains intact until a week later when the patient returns for suture removal.
- This is accomplished by gently lifting the edges of the film with a small forceps (*Fig. 76.5*).
- The sutures are nicely exposed and can be cut from this position.
- All the sutures can be removed en bloc by snipping them all and lifting off the film (which often includes hairs that have become embedded) (*Fig. 76.6*).

 Advantages:

- Bulky dressings are avoided.
- Patient can maintain normal hair style.

- While direct shampooing should be avoided, most patients can work around the wound area for grooming.

 Caveat:

- It is paramount to achieve complete hemostasis before the dressing is applied.

 Reference:

Salasche SJ. Surgical pearl: tips for scalp surgery. J Am Acad Dermatol 1994; 31:791–792.

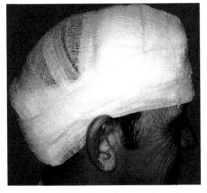

Fig. 76.1 Bulky head wrap dressing.

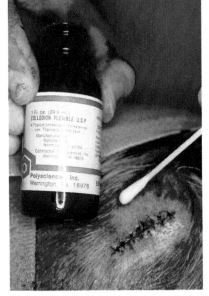

Fig. 76.2 Flexible collodion applied to a scalp wound.

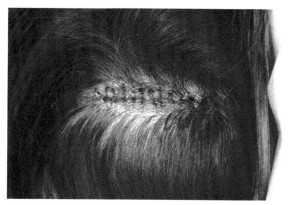

Fig. 76.3 Another wound showing the whitish film. (From Salasche SJ. Surgical pearl: tips for scalp surgery. J Am Acad Dermatol 1994; 31:791–792.)

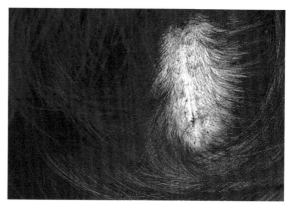

Fig. 76.4 After film and sutures removed en bloc.

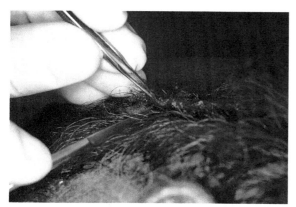

Fig. 76.5 Suture removal by lifting film from the side. (From Salasche SJ. Surgical pearl: tips for scalp surgery. J Am Acad Dermatol 1994; 31:791–792.)

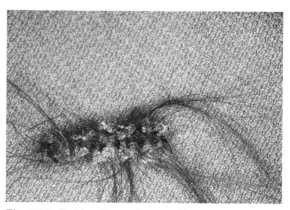

Fig. 76.6 En bloc film, sutures and hair.

Rationale:
- The lips and tongue are highly mobile and therefore difficult to stabilize during surgery.
- Below are some tips on how to overcome this.

 Technique:
- The simplest way to help immobilize and secure the tongue is with standard gauze sponges.
- Have the patient open their mouth and stick out their tongue.
- The tongue is then grasped gently with the sponges and held during the procedure (*Fig. 77.1*).
- A biopsy is required for a lesion on the upper surface of the mid-tongue (*Fig. 77.1*).
- After several minutes of topical application of a local anesthetic with viscous lidocaine on a cotton sponge, the patient is ready for local anesthesia.
- Immobilizing the tongue with the gauze sponge allows controlled injection of local anesthesia (*Fig. 77.2*).
- While waiting for the local anesthesia to take effect, the sponge is released and the patient is allowed to relax, close the mouth and swallow.
- Then, when the area is numb, with gauze immobilization the biopsy is performed (*Fig. 77.3*).
- Dental rolls help keep the field dry and the patient more comfortable.
- In this example, a shave biopsy has been done.
- If a punch biopsy were required, it would be better to pre-set one or two interrupted simple sutures around the intended biopsy site (*Fig. 77.4*).

- After the punch is performed, hemostasis is achieved with direct pressure with another gauze sponge.
- Finally, the pre-set stitches are tied (*Fig. 77.5*).
- 4-0 or 5-0 silk would be a good choice for suture material.
- Simple surgery on the lower lip can be facilitated by using a chalazion clamp, an instrument designed for the eyelid, but adaptable here.
- First attain anesthesia with a combination of regional mental nerve block and local infiltration with lidocaine containing epinephrine.
- The chalazion clamp is then applied, maintaining exposure of the surgical site (*Fig. 77.6*).
- Care must be taken not to ratchet down too tightly on the clamp and strangulate the lip.
- The clamp aids in stabilization as well as hemostasis (*Fig. 77.7*).

 Advantage:
- Simple methods of immobilizing and stabilizing the lip and tongue.

 Caveat:
- Avoid exerting too much pressure with the chalazion clamp; the mechanical advantage of the screw clamp is easy to underestimate.

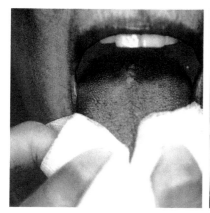

Fig. 77.1 Tongue held with gauze to expose leukokeratotic lesion.

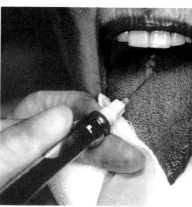

Fig. 77.2 Gauze-held tongue during local anesthesia.

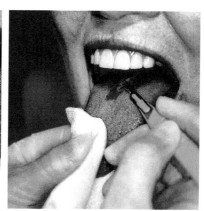

Fig. 77.3 Gauze-held tongue during shave biopsy.

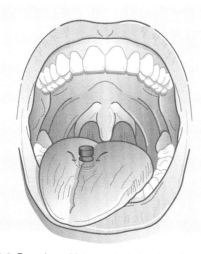

Fig. 77.4 Pre-placed interrupted simple suture under biopsy site.

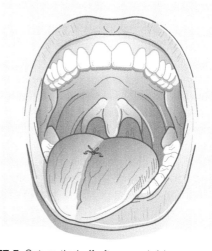

Fig. 77.5 Suture tied off after punch biopsy secured.

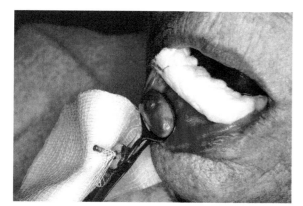

Fig. 77.6 Chalazion clamp aids removal of submucosal fibrosis.

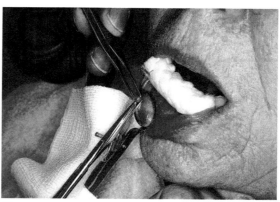

Fig. 77.7 Removal of submucosal fibrosis.

Suturing on the Lip to Minimize Patient Discomfort

Rationale:

- When nylon or absorbable sutures are used on the lip, the free edge and/or the knot of these sutures may be annoying to patients, particularly when talking or chewing.
- Some people actually lacerate their tongue by constantly licking the bristly stub of the exposed knot.
- Silk sutures are less irritating for the patient, but have the disadvantage of being more tissue reactive.
- If left in for more than a few days, silk incites sufficient inflammation and edema to make suture removal difficult.
- A simple modification of suturing technique will allow the surgeon to use nylon or other suture types without patient irritation.

Technique:

- Non-absorbable nylon or absorbable PDS, Dexon or Vicryl suture left over from the buried sutures may be used for the epidermal closure.
- A standard epidermal running suture is placed with its start point at the area most likely to get irritated, i.e. on the inner surface of the lip (Fig. 78.1).
- When the initial knot is tied, leave the free end approximately 1 cm long and 'tie it down' by securing it under the next several throws of the running suture (Figs 78.2, 78.3 and 78.4).
- Be sure this length of suture lies alongside the wound and not within it.
- If the end point of the running suture is also in an area that will be irritated, leave the free end here long also and then feed it back in and under the several previous throws of suture.

Advantages:

- This technique can prevent a very uncomfortable postoperative period for the patient.
- This allows sutures other than silk to be used for mucosal closures.
- Because the same suture used for the deep closure can be used, there is some cost savings.

Reference:

Fosko SW, Heap D. Surgical pearl: an economical means of skin closure with absorbable suture. J Am Acad Dermatol 1998; 39:248–250.

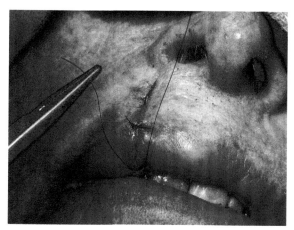

Fig. 78.1 Suturing begins intraorally, with end left long.

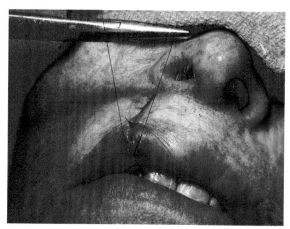

Fig. 78.2 Initial running mucosal suture bite. Free end held in position with hemostat by assistant.

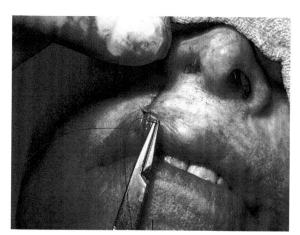

Fig. 78.3 Subsequent bites are placed in such a fashion as to wrap over the free short end with each successive throw.

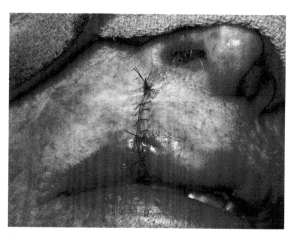

Fig. 78.4 Closure completed with the short end firmly secured under several throws of suture and incapable of causing irritation.

Labial Mucocele Removal

Rationale:

- Mucoceles are fluid-filled retention cysts of the mucosal lip due to injury of an underlying minor salivary gland (*Fig. 79.1*).
- They are usually asymptomatic, fluctuant nodules on the lower lip.
- They contain sialomucin.
- Treatments have included drainage and marsupialization, but excision remains the option least likely to result in a recurrence.

Technique:

- One method is to induce local anesthesia with a combination of a regional mental nerve block followed by local infiltration with lidocaine-containing epinephrine.
- A circumferential shallow incision is then made around the entire cyst but not into the cyst (*Fig. 79.2*).
- While stabilizing and pulling the lip away from the lesion on both sides, the index finger of one hand exerts upward pressure under the cyst to 'pouch' it out (*Fig. 79.3*).
- With a toothed forceps or a retraction suture to secure the mucosa over the cyst, the remainder of the cyst is separated off the underlying orbicularis oris muscle with a fine tissue scissors (*Fig. 79.4*).
- It is usually possible to deliver the cyst intact (*Figs 79.5 and 79.6*).
- The defect is then closed with an absorbable buried layer if there is significant dead space or simply closed on the surface with 5-0 silk sutures (*Fig. 79.7*).
- The silk sutures absorb fluid and remain soft and comfortable in the mouth.
- They can be removed in 4 or 5 days.

Variants:

- Others have placed retraction sutures into the mucosa at opposite ends of the cyst and intended line of excision.
- Using the two sutures for counter-traction, excision is carried out around the cyst down to the orbicularis oris muscle.

- A two-layered closure can be made using absorbable chromic or polyglactin with a superficial layer placed so that the knot is buried.
- The latter avoids irritating suture material in the mouth and precludes suture removal.

Advantages:

- Controlled excision with low recurrence incidence.
- Provides tissue for diagnosis confirmation.

Caveats:

- Care must be taken to know the projected pathway of the labial artery.
- If the artery is nicked or cut, a suture ligature must be placed on either side of the cut.

Reference:

Tran TA, Parlette HL. Surgical pearl: removal of a large labial mucocele. J Am Acad Dermatol 1999; 40:760–762.

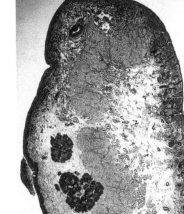

Fig. 79.1 The lip showing the minor salivary glands, the orbicularis oris muscle and the labial artery. (From Salasche SJ, Bernstein G, Senkarik M. Surgical Anatomy of the skin. Norwalk, Appelton and Lange, 1988.)

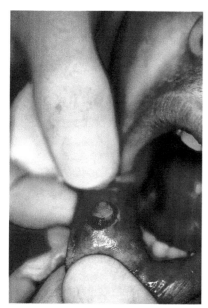

Fig. 79.2 Circumferential incision around the cyst.

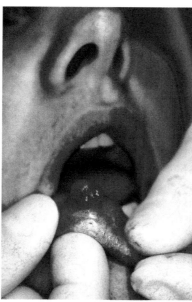

Fig. 79.3 Upward pressure pouches out the cyst.

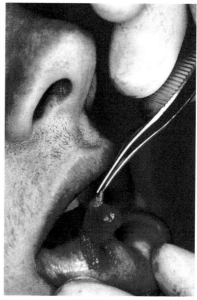

Fig. 79.4 Cyst held up by overlying mucus.

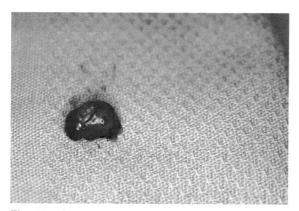

Fig. 79.5 Intact cyst.

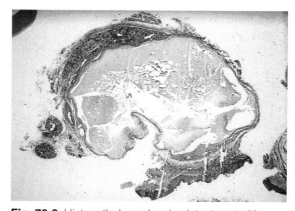

Fig. 79.6 Histopathology showing intact cyst with salivary glands on upper left and few orbicularis fibers on lower right.

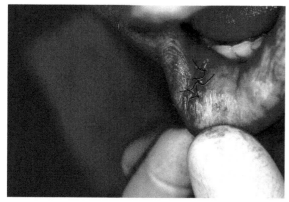

Fig. 79.7 Defect sewn shut with 5-0 silk sutures.

Dental Roll for Nasal Packing

 Rationale:
- Surgery of the nose is a common occurrence due to the disproportionate number of skin cancers that occur there.
- Dressings for the nose are usually custom designed for the individual, based on the size and location of the wound.
- Occasionally, surgery of the alar rim or around the nasal vestibule requires packing of the nares for support or to aid in hemostasis or graft survival.

 Technique:
- One indication for a nasal pack is to support a full-thickness skin graft of the ala nasi.
- If sufficient tissue depth is missing, it may be difficult to attain complete apposition of the wound bed to the undersurface of the graft with a standard pressure dressing (*Fig. 80.1*).
- Support can be attained by inserting a dental roll into the nostril (*Fig. 80.2*).
- This can be cut to just fit internally as well as end at the nasal vestibule (*Fig. 80.3*).
- This maneuver not only provides support but also helps immobilize the graft and aids in hemostasis during the critical first hours of graft take.

- The pack is left in place for 24 hours.
- Wrapping with petrolatum-impregnated gauze helps with insertion and removal.
- The packing may be crucial to graft survival (*Fig. 80.4*).
- Occasionally, a tumor may involve the alar base, nasal sill, the columella or the nasal vestibule.
- In this instance, the packing acts as a tamponade and aids hemostasis (*Figs 80.5, 80.6, 80.7 and 80.8*).

 Caveats:
- Advise patients that they may experience some degree of air hunger until they get used to the packing.
- It should not hurt and should be removed if it does become painful.
- Theoretically, it could form a nidus for infection, so it shouldn't remain in place for more than a day or two.

 References:

Winton GB, Salasche SJ. Wound dressings for dermatologic surgery. J Am Acad Dermatol 1985; 13:1026–1044.

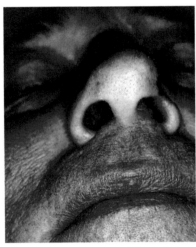

Fig. 80.1 Postsurgical defect of ala nasi with partially collapsed nares after placement of full-thickness skin graft.

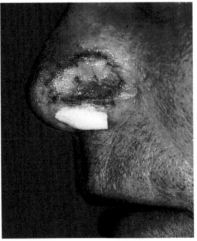

Fig. 80.2 Graft with dental roll in place.

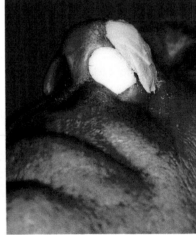

Fig. 80.3 Packing from basilar view.

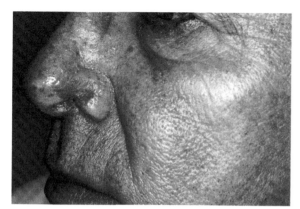

Fig. 80.4 Healing at 5 months.

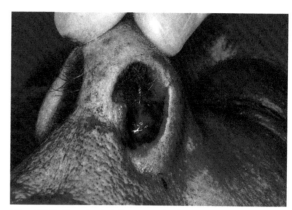

Fig. 80.5 Surgical defect on alar base mucosa.

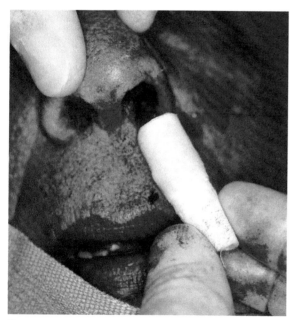

Fig. 80.6 Packing with petrolatum-impregnated gauze. (From Winton GB, Salasche SJ. Wound dressings for dermatologic surgery. J Am Acad Dermatol 1985; 13:1026–1044.)

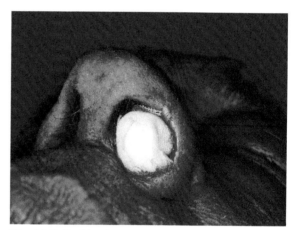

Fig. 80.7 Packing in place as tamponade. (From Winton GB, Salasche SJ. Wound dressings for dermatologic surgery. J Am Acad Dermatol 1985; 13:1026–1044.)

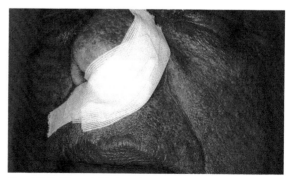

Fig. 80.8 Overnight dressing.

Rationale:
- Many surgical procedures are performed around the ear.
- This includes the temple, scalp and lateral cheek as well as the ear itself (*Figs 81.1 and 81.2*).
- Blood emanating from the wound may flow into and down the external auditory canal (*Fig. 81.3*).
- If blood dries on the tympanic membrane, it is irritating and also results in decreased auditory acuity by damping its vibratory ability.
- Removal may require installation of special dissolving fluids into the ear canal or even a visit to the otolaryngologist's office for manual flushing and removal.

Technique:
- Cotton balls may be placed in an individual instrument pack and gas sterilized.
- At the beginning of the procedure an appropriately sized bulky wad is placed comfortably into the external auditory canal (*Fig. 81.4*).
- It remains for the duration of the procedure, whereupon it can be removed after the final wound dressing is fashioned.
- Alternately, if there is continued drainage or as insurance against delayed bleeding, it may be left in place overnight (*Figs 81.5 and 81.6*).
- The patient is reminded to remove and discard the plug the next day.

Advantage:
- Prevents the problems enumerated above.

Caveats:
- Don't use a small plug or place it so deeply the patient has trouble removing it.
- Remind patient with the written wound care instructions to remove cotton the following day if the intent was to leave it in overnight.

References:
Salasche SJ, Winton GB, Adnot J. Surgical pearls. Dermatol Clin 1989; 7:75–110.

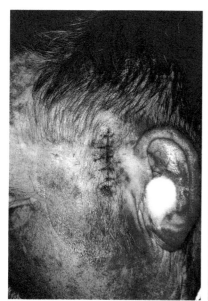

Fig. 81.1 Procedure in preauricular area.

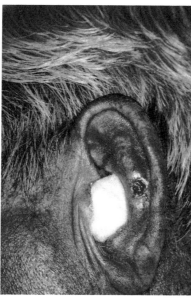

Fig. 81.2 Delayed repair of helix defect.

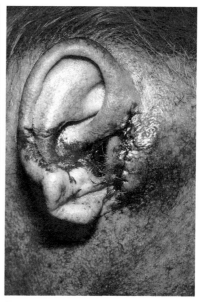

Fig. 81.3 Blood in canal from graft donor site wound.

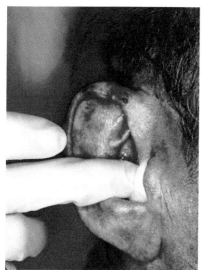

Fig. 81.4 Placement of cotton plug.

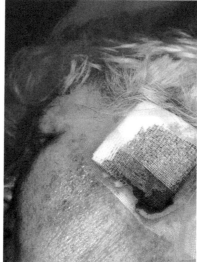

Fig. 81.5 Bleeding the night of surgery.

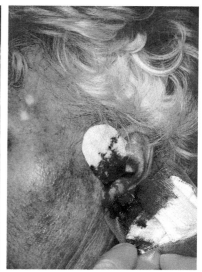

Fig. 81.6 Blood in canal with no cotton plug.

Rationale:

- The tension of wound closure for defects of the upper cheek or temple may impact negatively on the lower eyelid position.
- Even when the tension vector seems favorable, ultimate success depends on the relative ability of the lower eyelid to resist tension.
- As patients get older, loss of muscle strength and skin elasticity lessens the lid's ability to resist even minimum tension or weight.
- Wounds contract in all directions and have unexpected repercussions with on the final outcome.
- There is always the potential for function-impairing ectropion.
- Apposition of the inferior puncta to the globe of the eye is necessary for proper eye physiology.
- Ectropion leads to tearing (epiphora) and dry eye syndrome.
- So, when designing closures in this region, it is important to assess the integrity of the lower eyelid to try to anticipate unexpected problems.
- This includes both pre- and intraoperative assessments.

Technique:

- Preoperative assessment can be done with the 'snap' test (Fig. 82.1).
- The skin of the lower lid is grasped between the thumb and index finger and pulled away from the globe.
- In younger people the lid will snap back quickly to normal position. In older people, the lid may just 'ooze' slowly into place, indicating loss of lid strength integrity and an inability to withstand much tension or weight.
- Another preoperative assessment can be done with the 'tug' test (Fig. 82.2).
- The lower lid is tugged downward away from the globe with the surgeon's index finger.

- Assessing the resistance to the tugging gives similar information to the snap test.
- Little resistance should forewarn the surgeon that the lid will tolerate only minimal tension before it is displaced.
- Poor results from either test should be a warning to adjust the closure accordingly.
- Intraoperative assessment of the closure can be done by using instruments or a 'test' stitch to test the intended tension vector.
- An important maneuver is to have the patient sit up to a semi-reclining position and gaze upward with the mouth wide open (Figs 82.3 and 82.4).
- This stress maneuver reveals how the proposed closure will affect the eyelid after wound healing.

Advantages:

- Having the information from preoperative and intraoperative tests and maneuvers allows the surgeon to make good decisions.
- For the patient in Figures 82.7 and 82.8, it would be prudent to find another closure that redirects the tension vector to a more advantageous direction.
- Another example, (in Figures 82.5 and 82.6), where the stitches should be taken down and a more advantageous closure done. Off-set bias suturing may be the easiest solution (Tip 26).

Reference:

Salasche SJ. Complications of excisional and reconstructive surgery. In: Thiers BH, Lang PG, eds. Yearbook of dermatology and dermatologic surgery. St. Louis: Mosby; 2002:1–18.

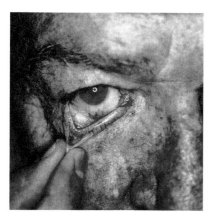

Fig. 82.1 The 'snap' test for eyelid strength.

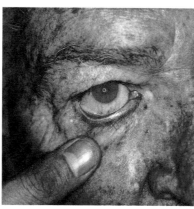

Fig. 82.2 The 'tug' test for eyelid strength.

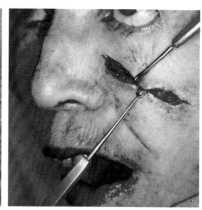

Fig. 82.3 Stress test with instruments. Note tension vector will not affect lower eyelid.

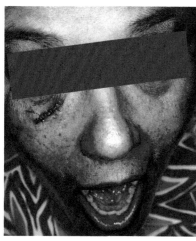

Fig. 82.4 Stress test after sutures placed; also no affect on lower lid.

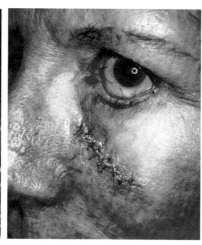

Fig. 82.5 Wound closure at repose.

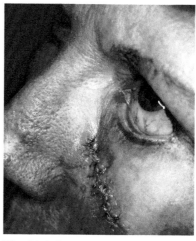

Fig. 82.6 Stress on wound closure reveals ectropion.

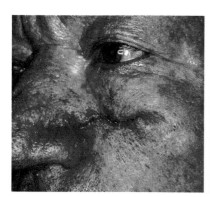

Fig. 82.7 Test stitch with vertical tension vector in repose.

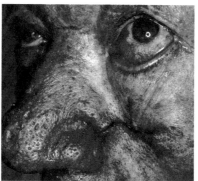

Fig. 82.8 Test stitch under stress unmasks ectropion.

Second-Intention Healing of Ear Defects

 Rationale:

- The ears are a frequent site of non-melanoma skin cancers.
- Because of the cartilage infrastructure of the ear, defects often require sophisticated repairs that involve tissue movement from the pre- or postauricular skin.
- Another approach is to temporize and allow initiation of healing by second intention to see if that approach will provide the best repair solution.
- Alternatively, the ensuing granulation and contraction may allow for the efficacious placement of a full-thickness skin graft or the ability to design a more simple flap.

 Technique:

- Defect after tumor extirpation of squamous cell carcinoma by Mohs micrographic surgery (*Fig. 83.1*).
- Note soft tissue involvement of helix, scapha, antihelix and triangular fossa.
- While there is some loss, for the most part the perichondrium and cartilage remain intact.
- Wound care consists of daily gentle cleansing and application of a moist, petrolatum-impregnated gauze.
- The patient is monitored at regular intervals to check on progress and possible alteration of the management plan if healing is not progressing satisfactorily.
- At 2 weeks, granulation and contraction are evident (*Fig. 83.2*).
- At 3 weeks, the helix has reshaped and the scapha and triangular fossa continue to fill in (*Fig. 83.3*).

- At 1 month, only the concavity of the scapha remains to heal.
- At 6 weeks, healing is complete with a final result that is certainly the match of a full-thickness skin graft (*Fig. 83.4*).

 Advantages:

- The patient is spared another procedure and its expense.
- If healing is monitored appropriately, surgical intervention is provided to prevent disfigurement that might lead to functional or cosmetic problems.

 Caveats:

- Patient selection is paramount.
- The cartilage and perichondrial cover should be mostly intact to provide an infrastructure and granulation tissue.
- As mentioned in Tip 81, a cotton wick in the external auditory canal during the first few days is a good precaution for preventing blood entering the canal and clotting on the tympanic membrane (see *Fig. 81.1*).
- Monitor for wound infections.
- While this rarely occurs, pseudomonas or other Gram-negative infections can be devastating.

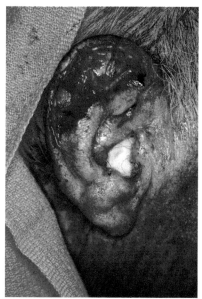

Fig. 83.1 Defect of upper anterior ear after tumor removal.

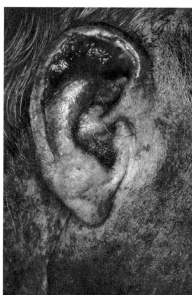

Fig. 83.2 Two weeks' healing by second intention.

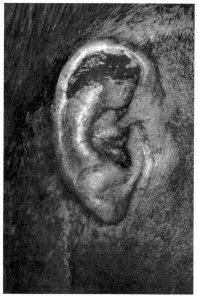

Fig. 83.3 Three weeks' healing.

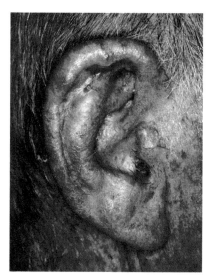

Fig. 83.4 Six weeks' healing.

Printed and bound by CPI Group (UK) Ltd, Croydon, CR0 4YY

03/10/2024

01040309-0020